ntial Guide to

nma

Catherine Short

Published in Great Britain in 2017 by

need2know

Remus House

Coltsfoot Drive

Peterborough

PE2 9BF

Telephone 01733 898103

www.need2knowbooks.co.uk

Contents

Introduction 7

Chapter 1: What is Asthma? 9

Definition 10
What are the symptoms? 10
What are the triggers? 11
Who is likely to develop asthma? 12
How is a diagnosis made? 12
Is asthma a serious condition? 13
What happens to my body when my asthma symptoms are troubling me? ... 14
What are inhalers and what do they do? 14
Summing Up 16

Chapter 2: Asthma Triggers 17

What is an asthma trigger? 18
What is an allergen? 18
Immunotherapy 21
What is allergy testing? 21
What is allergen avoidance? 21
What is allergen specific immunotherapy? 22
What is an exacerbation? 22
What about the future? 22
Summing Up 24

Chapter 3: Asthma Across the Ages 25

How is asthma diagnosed in younger children? 26
How do I find the right childcare? 27
School years – what about older children and teenagers? 28
Advice for teachers 29
What about adults with asthma? 30
What is occupational asthma? 30

How do hormone levels affect asthma in women? 32
How is asthma affected by puberty? 32
Will my asthma get worse during pregnancy and labour? 32
Will breastfeeding help my baby? 33
Will my asthma be affected by the menopause? 33
What are the special needs of the elderly? 34
What types of inhalers are more suitable for the elderly? 34
Summing Up 36

Chapter 4: Goals of Asthma Treatment 37

What are the goals of asthma treatment? 38
What are the treatments available and are they safe? 38
Short-acting bronchodilator therapy (Reliever therapy) 39
Inhaled corticosteroid therapy (Preventer therapy) 40
Long-acting bronchodilator therapy (Protector therapy) 41
Combination inhaler therapy 41
Leukotriene receptor antagonists 42
Steroid tablets 42
Theophylline tablets 43
Bronchodilator medicine 43
Compliance issues 43
Summing Up 45

Chapter 5: Types of Inhalers and Devices 47

Metered dose inhalers (MDI) 49
Turbohalers 50
Accuhaler inhaler 52
Autohalers 53
Easi-Breathe inhalers 54
Spacers/aerochambers 55
Nebulisers 56
Peak flow meters 57
Summing Up 59

Chapter 6: Smoking and Asthma 61

What are the effects of smoking on asthma? 62
Does smoking in pregnancy increase the risk of a baby developing asthma? 63
How does passive smoking affect us? 63
More reasons to stop smoking 64
Preparing to stop 65
Accessing help 66
Nicotine replacement therapy and other treatments explained 66
Summing Up 68

Chapter 7: How to Recognise and Manage an Attack 69

What are the reasons for sudden attacks? 70
How can I tell when an attack may be on the way? 71
What is the difference between an asthma attack and a panic attack? 73
Summing Up 76

Chapter 8: Making the Most of Your Review 77

What is the role of my general practitioner? 78
What is the role of the asthma nurse? 78
What should I expect from my asthma review? 80
What is self-management planning? 81
Why is inhaler technique so important? 81
What is influenza? 83
Pneumococcal vaccine 85
Summing Up 87

Chapter 9: Keeping Well 89

Stepping up and stepping down treatment – what does it mean? 90
How will I know that my asthma is poorly controlled? 92
What is airway remodelling? 93
Using a peak flow meter 93
Travel – thinking ahead 94
What is the role of rescue therapy? 95
Lifestyle advice 95
Allergen avoidance 95

Pre-Payment Certificates 96

Staying away from home overnight 96

Summing Up 98

Chapter 10: Additional Information **99**

Can complementary therapies help? 100

Can a nutritional approach help to control my asthma? 101

What are salicylates and how can they affect my asthma? 102

What is the 'Smart System'? 103

What are Xolair injections? 104

What is Bronchial thermoplasty? 104

Summing Up 105

Glossary **106**

Appendix A **108**

Appendix B **111**

Appendix C **114**

Help List **117**

Book List **120**

References and Bibliography **121**

Introduction

Asthma is a common condition causing inflammation, swelling, twitching, and thickening of the airways. The inflamed tissues also produce plugs of sticky mucus that is difficult to shift when you cough. This effect occurs in response to a wide range of triggers. Common triggers can include dust, animals, cold air, pollen and cigarette smoke. Asthma affects between 8 and 10% of children, and 5% of the adult population.

As the medical profession become more vigilant in looking for signs of this distressing and, sometimes fatal, condition, it is expected that numbers will continue to multiply. Asthma presents a huge burden on the purse strings of the National Health Service (NHS). Improving health education and care for sufferers will not only improve quality of life, reduce time off work and school and reduce preventable deaths from asthma, it will also reduce the financial burden on the NHS.

Are you persistently awoken during the night with breathlessness, coughing or wheezing? Have you had a troublesome cough in the middle of the night that may be linked with a recent general cold or flu-like illness? Do you have any of these symptoms, especially around hay fever season? Do you have a family history of asthma, especially on your mother's side of the family? If so, then you may suffer with asthma too.

> **Asthma affects between 8 and 10% of children, and 5% of the adult population.**

If you have already been given a diagnosis of asthma, you will probably have periods of time where you are unable to go to work or school and where you are sometimes limited in the amount of exercise you can do. Although there is no cure, understanding your condition, using modern treatment and following advice from your general practitioner (GP) or asthma nurse, there is no reason why you cannot enjoy a long, active and fulfilling life.

This informative, easy-to-read book is written for those who are affected by asthma, either newly diagnosed or long-term sufferers. If you are caring for a child or adult with asthma, then this book is also written with you in mind. Packed with the most up-to-date guidance and medical evidence available, this book will guide you through what asthma is, what the different kinds of inhalers are, how to use them correctly and explain how they work for you. We will look at other 'add-on' therapies that may need to be used in combination with your usual inhalers as well as common, age-specific problems and how to overcome them. The book also helps you to identify triggers and how to minimise exposure. One chapter is devoted to looking at the effects of cigarette smoking on asthma, including help and advice on where to go to get help if you want to stop smoking. You will also be able to use this book as an aid to asthma management, which should link in with guidance that may have been offered to you by a health-care professional.

Unfortunately, there are times when asthma can be troublesome, despite strict control. This self-help book will show you how to recognise early detection of poor control and how to manage it successfully. If you are unlucky enough to have a severe, sudden attack, this book will show you how to identify when you are in danger and provide you with the skills and confidence to manage your condition whilst seeking medical help. The aim of this book is to provide you with the tools and knowledge to help you gain control over your condition, rather than asthma taking control over you.

Acknowledgements

I would like to take this opportunity to thank those of you who have been so supportive and encouraging whilst I was writing this book. A huge thank you to Mandi Window my photographer, to nurse practitioner Sandra Gibbons, my proofreader and trusted friend. Thanks also to Professor David Garrod for your help and support. Special thanks to Asthma UK for all the information and for providing photos for my text. Thanks to Sally Welham at the British Thoracic Society and thank you to Chiesi Ltd for the wonderful photos.

Disclaimer

This book is for general information on asthma and isn't intended to replace professional medical advice. If you suspect that you have asthma, it is important to consult a health-care professional and obtain a proper diagnosis.

All the information in this book was correct at the time of going to press. National guidelines and recommendations can change, so it is important to check with your health-care professional before acting on any of the information in this book.

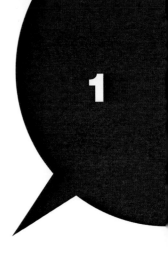

What is Asthma?

Definition

Asthma is defined as a chronic (long-term) inflammatory disorder of the airways, causing occasional (intermittent) obstruction to natural airflow, followed by periods of normal function. This is known as 'variability'. This inflammation causes swelling and twitchiness or irritability of the airways which then narrow as a response to common triggers.

Asthma can be either allergic or non-allergic (see chapter 2) and occurs more often in young male children. However, for older children and adults, it affects a greater number of females. More information on age-related problems is discussed in chapter 3.

The World Health Organisation (WHO) suggests that the number of asthma sufferers will continue to increase. One of the causative factors appears to be due to escalating numbers of house dust mite. It has been suggested that a decreased exposure to bacteria as a result of widespread prescribing of antibiotics, could be a significant contributing factor. Changes in diet and an increase in polyunsaturated fats are also attributed to increasing risk. A link to diesel fuels has been identified due to increased airborne pollution. Other causes have been identified, such as low birth weight, respiratory infections in infancy and early childhood, exposure to tobacco smoke, and dietary factors. Also, exercise, exposure to allergens, changes in weather, certain food additives and some medicines have been shown to trigger this unpredictable disease.

A genetic link has been identified, particularly on the maternal side, and this will be discussed more fully in chapter 3.

> **Asthma is defined as a chronic (long-term) inflammatory disorder of the airways, causing occasional (intermittent) obstruction to natural airflow, followed by periods of normal function.**

What are the symptoms?

Asthma symptoms include episodes of:

- Coughing.
- Tight chest.
- Wheezing.
- Shortness of breath.

As many suffers only ever cough, they do not realise that this symptom alone can be an identifying factor to asthma. These symptoms can often be worse at night or cause early morning waking. More rarely, asthmatics can experience chest pain, vomiting and itching, which are more commonly noticed in children.

Of course, any of these symptoms could be due to another cause, but your doctor or asthma nurse will be able to differentiate between asthma and other related conditions. Your doctor or nurse will ask you questions of when your symptoms started and what you were doing. The more information that you can give the doctor or nurse, the more effective their response will be in planning your individualised care plan.

What are the triggers?

As cited by Asthma UK, triggers are any thing or any substance which causes asthma symptoms to occur. Some common triggers are listed below, but we will look at these in more detail in chapter 2.

- Exercise can be a common trigger. Typically, a cough, wheeze or tight chest can occur twenty or thirty minutes after starting the exercise or occur after finishing your activity.

- Some children and adults will only develop symptoms after the onset of a cold. This viral infection can severely affect asthma.

- Temperature changes, particularly cold weather.

- House dust mite.

- Pollens.

- Animals, for example, cats, dogs, horses.

- Foods, such as peanuts, fizzy drinks and some alcohol.

- Aerosols, such as perfumes, deodorants and air fresheners.

- Excitement, laughter, emotional upset or stress.

- During hormonal surges, such as pregnancy, menopause or menstruation.

- Occupational asthma due to exposure to some chemicals.

It is important to remember that a trigger can cause a late response, up to twelve hours after exposure. Often, the late response can be much more severe.

As many suffers only ever cough, they do not realise that this symptom alone can be an identifying factor to asthma.

Who is likely to develop asthma?

Anyone can develop asthma, at any time of their life, but it does tend to run in families. Asthma is often linked with hay fever and eczema, so if these conditions run in your family, then you have a much greater chance of developing any one or all of them.

How is a diagnosis made?

Your doctor or asthma nurse will undertake what is termed a 'detailed history' in the form of asking you lots of questions about your symptoms, your family history, where you live, what your hobbies are, whether you have any pets, whether you are a smoker, if you are on any new medications.

Anyone can develop asthma, at any time of their life, but it does tend to run in families.

If you have suspected asthma, then your clinician may measure your 'peak expiratory flow rate' using a peak flow meter. This piece of equipment identifies obstruction in asthma. You will blow into this meter three times and the highest of the three readings will be recorded in your medical records. You may also be given an inhaler to use to help relieve your symptoms. You will then be asked to return to clinic a short while later. When you return, you will be asked about your response to the inhaler and the clinician will probably repeat the peak flow reading. With asthma, you often see a wide variation in the peak flow readings. This will help the doctor or nurse in determining your diagnosis and deciding if you need any additional inhalers. Using a peak flow meter will be explained more fully in chapter 5.

Sometimes, the nurse will perform a lung function test at the surgery called a 'spirometry test' where she may perform a 'reversibility test'. This involves performing a series of blows into the spirometer, and then having a number of puffs of an inhaler called Ventolin, through a device called a spacer. The blow test is then repeated fifteen minutes later. If there is a marked improvement in the readings following the Ventolin treatment, then the gap between the highest and lowest readings will demonstrate 'variability' or 'reversibility'. This is helpful in diagnosing asthma. The role of the doctor and nurse will be discussed more fully in chapter 8. Treatment options to help control your asthma will be discussed in detail in chapter 4.

Is asthma a serious condition?

Asthma can make sufferers seriously ill at times and, in some cases, it can kill. In 1997, it was estimated that there had been 27 deaths per million of the population in the UK, compared to 39 deaths per million in the late 1980s attributed to asthma.

Asthma is generally classified as intermittent, mild, moderate and severe. Most people fall into the mild to moderate category for asthma. It can also become dormant for long periods of time and then be triggered through stages in life such as pregnancy, menopause or old age. More worryingly, some people who appear to have dormant asthma can, without warning, develop severe asthma. In my experience, people with severe asthma attend the surgery in clusters, around April, due to pollen activity. Then September/October, due to the mushroom and mould development. And again in the winter months as a result of worsening asthma, triggered by a common cold or flu-like illness.

Identifying and understanding your symptoms is key to learning how to recognise if your asthma is worsening. Identifying and managing a severe attack will be looked at in more detail in chapter 7.

In 1997, it was estimated that there had been 27 deaths per million of the population in the UK, compared to 39 deaths per million in the late 1980s attributed to asthma.

What happens to my body when my asthma symptoms are troubling me?

As mentioned earlier, asthma is characterised by episodes of obstruction and narrowing within the airways. Increased reactivity of the airways can result from breathing in irritants or being exposed to a trigger, which in turn, cause inflammation.

The walls of the main airways, the main bronchus and bronchioles, are made up of muscle tissue, connective tissue, goblet cells and mucus glands. The mucus glands line the surface of the airway and secrete mucus. Goblet cells also produce mucus. During an asthmatic episode, the smooth muscle fibres become twitchy and contract, causing shorter, narrower airways. This produces spasm and symptoms of a tight chest. The secretory cells produce thick, sticky secretions that form plugs of mucus which further block the airways.

The inflammation in the airways causes further swelling as a result of increased localised blood flow. This further reduces the lumen (the space through which the air flows within the airways) causing further obstruction.

What are inhalers and what do they do?

Your doctor or asthma nurse will have arranged a prescription for inhalers. Depending on how badly affected you are by your asthma, your health-care professional will choose one or more inhalers suitable for you. We shall look at the different inhalers briefly here, although they will be discussed in more detail in chapters 4 and 5.

The main groups of inhalers are:

- Relievers, which immediately relax the smooth muscle fibres, allowing the spasm to settle. The effect begins to take place as soon as you use the inhaler with maximum effect after fifteen minutes. These reliever inhalers are nearly always blue. This is the inhaler that you would use when you become symptomatic and it will settle your symptoms quickly.

- Preventers are inhalers which contain low dose corticosteroids (steroids), which act as an anti-inflammatory agent. These mop up the inflammation and if the dose is correct, this will control your asthma. This is commonly termed 'good control'. It generally takes about two weeks for the preventer inhaler to become effective. Therefore, this inhaler is never used in an emergency. These inhalers tend to be brown, burgundy or orange.

- Protector inhalers are added to preventer therapy when the preventor is not efficient enough to reduce your symptoms fully. These are called 'long acting bronchodilators' and they relax the smooth muscle walls for twelve hours at a time. They usually take more than twenty minutes before they begin to work, so they would never be used in an emergency. These inhalers are often green.

- Combination inhalers are useful to use if you need to take a preventer and a protector each day. Combining the inhalers reduces the number of inhalers that you need to use. As mentioned previously, these contain inhaled corticosteroid mixed with a long acting bronchodilator. These inhalers are often purple or red.

- Leukotriene receptor antagonists are tablets taken at night when further improvement is needed. They are particularly good for exercise and allergy-induced asthma symptoms. These have been found to be very useful, particularly for children where symptomatic control has been difficult to establish.

- Steroid tablets are used when your asthma is severe. They are added to the above treatments and are taken first thing in the morning. They act by reducing the inflammation very quickly and become effective usually after eight hours of taking.

If you need to use your blue inhaler more than three times per week, or if you are waking at night due to your asthma, it is time to make an appointment to see your doctor or asthma nurse.

Summing Up

- Your asthma is a long-term condition, but it needn't control your life. With careful self-management under the guidance of your doctor or nurse, asthma can be successfully managed.

- Asthma symptoms include a wheeze, a cough, shortness of breath and a tight chest, but it is important to remember that you may not have all of these symptoms.

- Think about what your triggers may be and see if there are any ways that you can avoid them. Don't forget the delayed onset of symptoms, which can be up to twelve hours after exposure to your trigger.

- Anyone can develop asthma at any stage in their life, but is often linked with a strong family history of atopy, or in other words, a family history linked to allergic conditions.

- Your doctor or asthma nurse will diagnose your asthma.

- The asthmatic response causes twitchiness and contraction of the muscle fibres. Inflammation causes swelling of the tissues and increased production of thick mucus including sticky plugs. Both of which make it harder to breathe.

- Asthma is classified as intermittent, mild, moderate or severe.

- Your usual inhaler will be a reliever which offers immediate relief. You may also need a preventer inhaler to dampen down the inflammation. Sometimes a long acting bronchodilator needs to be added too.

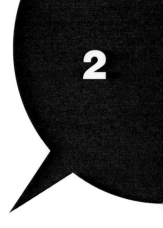

Asthma Triggers

What is an asthma trigger?

An asthma trigger is anything that can cause the inflammation of the airways, leading to the symptoms of coughing, wheezing or shortness of breath that you normally would associate with asthma. Your triggers can be numerous and varied. They can be in the form of an allergen or an environmental exposure to an irritant.

Some important research has shown that when hay fever (allergic rhinitis) and asthma co-exist, treating the hay fever with nasally inhaled steroids can effectively control the asthma at the same time.

What is an allergen?

This is any substance that causes an allergic reaction in a person sensitive to it.

As mentioned in chapter 1, common triggers in this group are:

- House dust mite along with pet dander (material shed from an animal's coat) – This is one of the most common airborne allergens.

- Pollens – More commonly grass and tree pollen. Asthma and hay fever (allergic rhinitis) often co-exist and hay fever alone can be an independent risk factor in the development of asthma. Hay fever suffers frequently complain of clear nasal discharge, itching, watery eyes and a stuffed up nose, which is accompanied by sneezing. These symptoms can begin as early as February, when the tree pollens first appear. If you or your child have asthma and hay fever simultaneously, then this can cause worsening symptoms. Interestingly, some important research has shown that when hay fever (allergic rhinitis) and asthma co-exist, treating the hay fever with nasally inhaled steroids can effectively control the asthma at the same time.

- Moulds – The effect of inhaling them can cause severe symptoms, particularly during the autumn months when fungus and mushrooms can be found. Rotting leaves and plants can have an unsettling effect on asthma.

- Pet dander – Even something as lovely as visiting grandparents can be troublesome if you or your child are allergic to Granny's pet dog or cat. Interestingly, you can become desensitised to your own pet. Unfortunately, if your pet dies and is replaced, this can set off your symptoms all over again. Some people are allergic to horses too. If you or your child are allergic to a pet, even though this is deeply distressing, you will need to consider removing the pet from the home. Despite this, it can take up to six months for the allergens to fall sufficiently to provide a reduction in symptoms.

- Cigarette smoke – This has been identified as one of the most common asthma irritants. Mothers smoking during pregnancy increase the risk of the baby developing asthma. Smoking during the postnatal period exposes the baby to smoke and increases the risks. Smoking-related asthma will be discussed more fully in chapter 6.

- Foodstuffs – Peanuts, alcohol and food additives can affect asthma. Peanuts are a particular problem as they can bring on a life-threatening effect called 'anaphylactic shock' which is always a medical emergency. Those people who know that they have had this type of severe allergic reaction before, often carry what is called an 'EpiPen'. This injectable, pen-like device delivers a shot of adrenaline which controls the allergic reaction, while waiting for an ambulance. These people should always carry two EpiPens. A second dose can be administered five minutes later if the ambulance is delayed. This special treatment is prescribed by a general practitioner (GP). If you or your child needs to carry this treatment, then book an appointment with your practice nurse, where she can show you how to use it safely and effectively.

- Emotions – For example, laughter, stress and excitement can all bring on asthma symptoms. If I watch a funny film or laugh a lot, I find that I can cough for ages afterwards, which drives my husband mad!

- Aerosols, perfumes and deodorants, and air fresheners – these can trigger your asthma.

- Some medicines, such as aspirin, non-steroidal anti-inflammatories, and Timoptol eye drops – These can exacerbate asthma symptoms. Unfortunately, these symptoms can be delayed and very severe too.

- Occupational asthma due to chemicals – Once this diagnosis has been confirmed, measures need to be put into place to remove the person from exposure. If possible, relocation away from exposure should occur within twelve months of the first identified work-related symptoms. Prematurely changing your occupation is not advised at this stage. This will be discussed more fully in chapter 3.

- Air pollution – Evidence has shown that due to the high diesel particulate environment, asthma and allergy is on the increase. Air pollution has been found to provoke asthma attacks or aggravate current disease levels and it can result in changes in the numbers of hospital admissions due to asthma exacerbations.

- Extremes of temperature – Extremes, particularly cold air, can trigger asthma symptoms.

- The common cold virus – Colds and other upper respiratory tract infections such as flu, sinusitis, and sore throats can all trigger susceptible asthmatics. This can occur one or two days after the virus causes symptoms, so not only do you have a nasty cold, but your cough, wheeze, chest tightness or shortness of breath can be worsened due to your asthma. This can sometimes trigger a severe exacerbation of asthma.

- Exercise-induced asthma – This is a common trigger, especially in children. If this is a recognised trigger, it is important that you or your child have adequate treatment which enable him or her to participate fully in any sport. This is achievable and is termed 'optimal control'. In other words, treat the asthma rather than stop the activity. It is important to encourage exercise in children.

Asthma is often classified into two groups:

Atopic asthma or extrinsic asthma

Up to 50% of sufferers can also have symptoms of other similar conditions such as hay fever and eczema.

This form of asthma is typically associated with allergy. An allergic reaction occurs when a specific allergen comes into contact with someone who is sensitive to the substance. If you are atopic, it means that you have a pre-disposition to developing allergic conditions such as asthma, hay fever and eczema. Being atopic doesn't necessarily cause these conditions, but it does make you more susceptible to developing them. Therefore, allergens can trigger allergic reactions in susceptible people. Up to 50% of sufferers can also have symptoms of other similar conditions such as hay fever and eczema. They also have high levels of an immunoglobulin E (IgE) in their bloodstream. This antibody has been identified as a general marker for allergic conditions. Often, a strong family history can be found.

Non-atopic asthma or intrinsic asthma

'IgE antibodies are produced in response to contact with normally harmless substances. This is known as sensitisation. Once this has happened, further exposure to the same substance will lead to an immune reaction, causing symptoms in the affected person.'

Allergy Week – Special Edition April 2011, Allergy UK.

This pattern of asthma is more common where someone has developed adult onset asthma. The symptoms are more persistent in comparison to atopic asthma. Often a trigger cannot be identified.

Immunotherapy

This is sometimes considered in people with asthma where an allergen cannot be avoided. This treatment can be dangerous with the potential for a severe allergic reaction. If your GP suspects that you or your child would benefit from immunotherapy, these considerations would be fully discussed with a specialist first.

What is allergy testing?

This is a useful test in helping to identify common triggers to enable you or your child to avoid any allergens that you can, in order to reduce symptoms. It involves a specially trained clinician who will discuss the symptoms and triggers through a detailed allergy history. This information is useful in combination with skin prick tests and blood testing for IgE levels, which all assist in the identification of specific allergens or sensitisation. This enables you or your child to reduce exposure to a specific allergen.

What is allergen avoidance?

If you or your child are allergic to the most common allergen, house dust mite, then it is important to reduce exposure. This needs commitment from all the family and involves:

- Special bedding protection.

- Carpets replaced with wooden floor or laminated flooring.

- Soft toys being put in plastic bags and frozen for 6-8 hours which will kill the dust mites. The toy is then defrosted.

- Bed linen washed at high temperatures (above 60°C).

- The use of a dehumidifier can be effective.

If you or your child is allergic to the most common allergen, house-dust mite, then it is important to reduce exposure. This needs commitment from all the family.

Even with rigorous measures, total relief of symptoms is not possible and at best, you will only reduce the severity of the condition. A group of independent experts called 'The Cochrane Collaboration' looked at 54 differing trials which compared chemical and physical methods of mite avoidance. They found that these methods failed to be effective and they did not recommend this practice. However, this is not to say that it is not important to reduce known triggers, as increased exposure can lead to worsening of symptoms and a deterioration in lung function. Over time, deterioration may become irreversible, leading to chronic or long-term lung disease.

What is allergen specific immunotherapy?

This is a procedure where a known allergen is injected under the skin of a sufferer and it has been found to reduce asthma symptoms and the use of asthma medication. It has also been shown to improve the sensitivity of the lungs. However, it is not without risk. The Cochrane Collaboration (a group of experts who provide high quality evidence) has cited that it does increase risk of severe and fatal anaphylaxis.

What is an exacerbation?

Sudden worsening of asthma called 'asthma exacerbations' often occur in seasonal cycles, triggered during the winter by the cold and flu season, as a result of a viral infection, or triggered through exposure to pollens, dusts and seasonal moulds. Also, an exacerbation in children can be amplified during a cough or cold, due to poor air quality and exposure to allergens. Identification and management of an asthma exacerbation will be discussed fully in chapter 7.

What about the future?

Pioneering work at the University of Manchester suggests that allergic conditions such as asthma, eczema and hay fever could be a thing of the past.

This exciting treatment will take the form of special drugs that will stop the allergens from entering the body, therefore eradicating the effect of the allergen. These drugs are called 'allergen delivery inhibitors'. They work by blocking the ability of the allergen from entering through skin and lung tissue and blocking the allergic reaction before it occurs.

If found to be effective, these drugs will be used to treat symptoms in adult sufferers and then could be used to prevent allergies in children.

Summing Up

- An asthma trigger is any allergen or environmental factor which irritates the airways, causing symptoms associated with asthma such as a cough, a wheeze or shortness of breath.

- Asthma is classified into two groups – atopic and intrinsic asthma.

- Allergy testing is useful in identifying common triggers and is undertaken through a detailed allergy history, a skin prick test and a blood test.

- Allergen avoidance means reducing exposure to a known trigger. This helps to reduce the frequency and severity of your asthma symptoms.

- Allergen Specific Immunotherapy involves the injection of a known allergen under the skin with the goal of reducing sensitivity to the trigger. But it can be risky in terms of a severe or life-threatening reaction.

- An asthmatic exacerbation is a sudden worsening of symptoms due to a severe reaction to a trigger and it can be life-threatening.

Asthma Across the Ages

Did you know that boys are three times more likely to be affected before puberty compared to girls? Interestingly, prevalence is equal between boys and girls by adolescence. Adult-onset asthma is more common in women and the rise in females developing asthma has been linked to puberty.

How is asthma diagnosed in younger children?

Did you know that boys are three times more likely to be affected before puberty compared to girls?

Diagnosis in children under the age of six is difficult. Interestingly, wheezing is not always as a result of asthma and can be due to other causes. In the under twos, common reasons for wheezing include bronchiolitis and wheezy bronchitis. Also, in rare circumstances, a wheeze can indicate that a child has inhaled a foreign body, such as a small toy.

At least one child in seven will suffer with a wheeze-type episode at some point during the first five years of life, and many of these children will not go on to develop asthma in later childhood. For this reason, your doctor or asthma nurse may be reluctant to give a formal diagnosis of asthma.

Your doctor or nurse will look at the pattern of symptoms over time before diagnosing asthma. He/she will take a detailed history and will listen carefully to the story that you tell regarding your child's symptoms. Included in this will be any asthma links to others in the family and whether your child has any other allergic (atopic) symptoms such as hay fever or eczema. If this detailed history suggests that your child has probable asthma, the nurse or doctor may prescribe what is called a 'trial of treatment' of a bronchodilator. They may also include a steroid inhaler at this stage, depending on the severity and frequency of your child's symptoms.

Your child and the effectiveness of the treatment will be closely monitored. You will probably be asked to keep a record of your child's symptoms and when they occur. This will give your doctor or asthma nurse very useful information in helping determine the cause of symptoms. If your child responds well to the treatment and the reliever offers effective relief of symptoms, then this will offer a probable asthma diagnosis. If the treatment is not effective then this will suggest a different cause for their symptoms, where referral to a specialist may be necessary.

For adults and children over the age of six, the diagnosis is made much easier with the help of equipment such as a spirometer or peak flow meter (as discussed in chapter 1) which will be able to demonstrate 'variability' or 'reversibility' which is a clear indicator of asthma. The lung function tests are very effort-dependent and so some children are unable to perform the tests effectively and accurately. The treatments and inhalers will be discussed more fully in chapters 4 and 5.

Generally speaking, some children with asthma appear to lose their symptoms when they reach adulthood and others may find their symptoms are milder. Recent research shows that asthma can lay dormant for long periods of time, almost as if the condition has disappeared. However, the symptoms may return in later life.

'In trying to establish a diagnosis in children, health professionals often depend on the parent's description of symptoms. However, some parents are unclear what wheeze sounds like, and mistake noisy breathing from upper airway secretions...'

Mark Levy, Linda Pearce, *Asthma*, Mosby, 2004.

How do I find the right childcare?

This is often a daunting task for any parent which can be increasingly more worrying when your child has asthma.

Here are three key questions that you might like to consider when seeking childcare:

1 Does the childminder or nursery have an asthma policy?

2 Are they able to provide care for your child when he/she is having problems?

3 Do they know how to recognise and deal with an asthmatic emergency?

Asthma UK suggest that all childcarers and nurseries should have an asthma policy in place which should cover:

- The environment your child will be in.

- The training that a carer has received if they intend to give your child their asthma treatment when it is needed.

Generally speaking, some children with asthma appear to lose their symptoms when they reach adulthood and others may find their symptoms are milder.

- How they would proceed during an asthma emergency.

- The environment should be safe, where triggers will be avoided and where asthma inhalers are easily accessible to be used under supervision.

- Your child's carer should be able to identify when your child is having an asthma attack and know how to deal with this.

Once you have chosen your child's carer, provide them with written details of:

- Your child's asthma therapy and how and when to take them.

- All emergency contact phone numbers.

- Information of any known triggers that aggravate your child's asthma.

Ensure that all your child's inhalers are clearly labelled with your child's name, that your child's carer has spares and that the expiry dates on the medication are checked regularly.

If your child is more affected than usual or if he/she is symptomatic during the night, tell your child's carer so that she can keep a close eye on him/her.

School years – what about older children and teenagers?

There are approximately two children per classroom in the UK who have asthma.

Interestingly, only 65% of parents are confident that their child's PE teacher knows how to manage their child's condition during an asthma attack.

It is important that you develop a good working partnership with your child's school and that you feel confident that the school is able to care for your child's needs.

Advice for parents:

- Tell the school that your child has asthma.

- Ensure that the school has up-to-date written information about all your child's medicines and inhalers, how much they will need and when. This could take the form of a 'written self-management plan' that could be written in partnership with your asthma nurse. Also, try and include information about your child's known triggers.

Ensure that the school has up-to-date written information about all your child's medicines and inhalers, how much they will need and when. This could take the form of a written self-management plan' that could be written in partnership with your asthma nurse. Also, try and include information about your child's known triggers.

- If your child attends visits, field trips or sporting activities away from school whilst under the supervision of the school, ensure that the teacher taking the group has access to up-to-date information regarding medicines and inhalers that may need to be taken.

- Inform the school of any changes in your child's asthma, particularly if they are getting more frequent symptoms or are waking frequently at night.

- Make sure that the school has a spare inhaler for your child to use and that it is in date. Ensure it is labelled with your child's name.

- Keep your child off school if they are unwell, particularly if they have been troubled by symptoms at night.

- Ensure that your child is given extra support from school to catch up on missed lessons.

- Make sure that your child has access to their inhaler at all times.

- Find out if there will be any problems getting access to inhalers during break and dinner time. Are the dinner ladies aware of asthma management?

- Always remember that if your child's asthma has become troublesome, make an appointment to see your asthma nurse or doctor. Prompt action may prevent a severe attack.

Advice for teachers

- You can help parents of children with asthma too. If you notice that the child in your class is coughing, breathless or wheezing, particularly during sport, it may be a good idea to let the parents know. They may not be aware and this will help prompt a visit to the nurse or doctor for a review.

- The more access to information that you have, the more this will ultimately help the child in your care. Inhaler technique is most important and if you are aware of these issues, you can feed back to parents if you are concerned that the child is not managing his/her inhaler. Asthma UK has an excellent website, where a simple, yet excellent video of inhaler technique can be found.

- It is important that both parents are equally involved and informed in their child's healthcare, especially if the child is co-parented.

- Remember that, by working in partnership with parents, the child in your care will have a better school attendance if their asthma is well controlled. If you are concerned, you may wish to ask the child's parents if the child is symptomatic at home, especially during the night.

- Your school nurse will also be an excellent resource and will be able to help answer any of your questions, or will be able to refer you to someone who can help.

What about adults with asthma?

Asthma is mostly considered a childhood complaint, yet there are some people who develop symptoms later in life. This is termed 'adult-onset asthma'.

In adults, symptoms are often triggered by:

- Flu, coughs, sore throats – often viral infections.

- Laughing or extremes of emotion.

- Exercise. Symptoms usually appear twenty or thirty minutes into the episode or at the end.

- Times of anxiety or depression.

- Some medicines such as aspirin, ibuprofen, naproxen, Timoptol eye drops, beta blockers.

- Inhalation of cigarette smoke, aerosols such as perfumes, air fresheners, deodorants.

Other conditions that mimic asthma include: bronchitis, emphysema, heart disease and chronic obstructive airways disease. All of these conditions complicate the diagnosis of asthma.

What is occupational asthma?

The Health and Safety Executive estimates that between 1,500 and 3,000 adults in the UK develop occupational asthma each year. The condition can take weeks or years to become obvious. The substances that cause asthma are called 'respiratory sensitisers' and currently, over 200 sensitisers have been identified.

High-risk occupations include:

The Health and Safety Executive estimates that between 1,500 and 3,000 adults in the UK develop occupational asthma each year.

need2know

- Bakers and pastry makers.

- Spray painters, welders and solderers.

- Laboratory animal workers.

- Health care workers and dental carers.

- Metalworkers and woodworkers.

- Chemical and food processors.

- Texttile, plastics and rubber manufacturers.

- Cleaners and hairdressers.

- Farmers and other occupations where there is risk of exposure to fumes and dust.

If you think that your job is affecting your asthma, look out for these common signs:

- Your asthma is worse during your working week and you feel better at weekends.

- Your symptoms settle when you are away from work, such as when you are on holiday.

Did you know that there was up to 1.1 million lost working days due to breathing or lung conditions during 2008/09?

Did you know that you could be at risk of developing asthma through the job that you do?

Were you aware that your job could be causing new triggers for your asthma while you are at work?

Advice for colleagues:

If you are concerned about a colleague's health and are worried that it is occupation related, speak to them about it. If they agree that there may be a problem, then encourage your colleague to speak to the health and safety leader, or your manager.

How do hormone levels affect asthma in women?

Normal cyclical hormonal levels that change during puberty, menstruation, pregnancy and the menopause can all affect your asthma.

How is asthma affected by puberty?

Adolescent girls with asthma can have episodes of poor control, due to the influences of hormones during puberty. Asthma can become worse when a girl begins menstruating for the first time. Once menstruation becomes regular, asthma usually settles down. Even so, one third of females become symptomatic pre-menstrually or during their period. This can be managed by increasing your preventer inhaler the week prior to your period, but speak to your asthma nurse first. Don't forget to do your peak flow readings and take them to your appointment.

Paracetamol for period pain is safe and doesn't affect your asthma, but be careful with non-steroidal, anti-inflammatories such as naproxen, Nurofen, ibuprofen and Ponstan, as this group of drugs can worsen your asthma.

> Hormonal changes can affect asthma in adolescent girls. Some girls find their asthma is worse around the time their periods start for the first time.

Will my asthma get worse during pregnancy and labour?

Many women worry about the effects of their asthma therapy during pregnancy and labour. Interestingly, one third of women find their asthma improves during pregnancy, while one third stay the same and the other third become more symptomatic. It is important that you seek advice if your asthma is troubling you during pregnancy. Your baby will develop normally if you are under control and breathing normally.

- Inhaled medicines are safe for your baby.

- There is no convincing evidence to support the idea that avoiding certain foods will reduce the chance of your baby developing asthma. Despite this, women who are pregnant and have immediate family members with asthma, hay fever and eczema, are advised to avoid any foods containing peanuts during pregnancy and breastfeeding.

- During labour, your body produces increased levels of natural steroid hormones such as adrenaline and cortisone. These increased levels have a protective effect in terms of asthma, during labour.

- If you still have trouble during labour, you will be able to use your usual reliever inhaler, as it will not be harmful to your baby.

- Take into account your asthma when you draw up your birthing plan with your midwife or doctor. Any worries can be discussed then.

- There is more risk of an infant developing asthma if they are premature or with a low birth weight, or if you smoked during pregnancy. Also, smoking during pregnancy increases your baby's risk of being wheezy or having breathing problems. There is a 35% chance that your child will develop asthma if you smoke during pregnancy.

- Acute asthma is rare during labour. You should continue your usual inhalers during pregnancy and labour and your baby will not be affected by your normal asthma therapy during breastfeeding.

There is a 35% chance that your child will develop asthma if you smoke during pregnancy.

Will breastfeeding help my baby?

- Some studies have suggested that if you breastfeed your baby for the first few months of life, you will reduce your baby's chances of developing allergic conditions including asthma, hay fever and eczema.

- Your normal inhaled asthma therapy will not harm your baby in any way. Also, it will not affect your ability to breastfeed or your ability to produce milk. There will be no traces of the inhaled medicine in the breast milk.

- Evidence also shows that infants are offered some protection in developing asthma if they are breastfed.

Will my asthma be affected by the menopause?

At this time in a woman's life, there are marked hormonal changes which can influence your asthma. It may improve or become more troublesome. If you are troubled by regular symptoms, remember to keep your peak flow diary and take your readings to your appointment with your asthma nurse/doctor.

What are the special needs of the elderly?

For those who have suffered with asthma most of their life, when they reach old age, their triggers can change. Also, their symptoms may change too. They may have coughed or wheezed when they were younger, but they may, as they get older, become more breathless.

Common triggers for the elderly include:

- Flu and colds and other viral infections.
- Exercise.
- Laughter and extremes of emotion.
- Some medicines.
- Anxiety or depression.
- Cigarette smoke.
- Perfumes and chemical fumes.

Some people are diagnosed with asthma late in life. This is called "late-onset asthma". Of those that develop asthma later in life, 70% do not have an allergic cause.

Some people are diagnosed with asthma late in life. This is called 'late-onset asthma'. Of those that develop asthma later in life, 70% do not have an allergic cause. So, in this age group, it is less likely that asthma is triggered by allergens such as house dust mite, feathers, furry animals and pollen.

Sometimes other conditions can mimic asthma, such as heart disease, chronic obstructive pulmonary disease (COPD), chronic bronchitis and emphysema. This makes a diagnosis more difficult. Visit your GP or practice nurse to start on the road to a correct diagnosis.

What types of inhalers are more suitable for the elderly?

As we get older, our manual dexterity can worsen, often due to joint changes, neurological changes and sight problems. For this reason, elderly asthmatics may struggle to use their usual inhalers, causing inhaler technique to worsen which ultimately reduces the effectiveness of their inhaled medication. If you are elderly or you look after someone who is, and you are worried about technique, this is an excellent opportunity to prompt a visit to your asthma nurse or doctor. Please make sure you take your usual inhalers to the appointment, where the nurse or doctor can check inhaler technique.

The speed at which someone can draw in their usual inhaled therapy through their usual device is called 'inspiratory flow rate'. As we get older, our inspiratory flow rate reduces and this sometimes means that we need to change to a different type of inhaler to improve absorption. Differing inhalers will be discussed more fully in chapter 5.

Summing Up

- Diagnosis of asthma under the age of six is difficult. A detailed history and monitoring the effectiveness of inhalers will aid diagnosis.

- Ensure that your childminder's or nursery's asthma policy is up to date and that they know how to deal with your child's condition.

- Encourage effective communication with your child's teachers in order to ensure that your child's asthma is as well controlled as possible. This will reduce days off school due to illness related to asthma.

- If you are a teacher of an asthmatic child, make sure you let the child's parents know if their child is more symptomatic during your care.

- If you develop adult-onset asthma, it may be linked to your occupation.

- Normal hormonal, cyclical changes in women can affect asthma during puberty, menstruation, pregnancy, lactation and the menopause.

- Reduced manual dexterity due to age can interfere with inhaler technique.

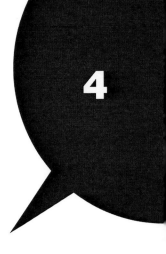

4

Goals of Asthma Treatment

Sadly, an estimated 75% of hospital admissions for asthma are avoidable and as many as 90% of the deaths from asthma are preventable. The NHS spends around one billion pounds a year treating and caring for people with asthma.

What are the goals of asthma treatment?

'The aim of pharmacological management of asthma is the control of symptoms, including nocturnal symptoms and exercise-induced asthma, prevention of exacerbations and the achievement of best possible pulmonary function, with minimal side effects.'

Thorax - an International Journal of Respiratory Medicine - British Guidelines on the Management of Asthma. BMJ Publishing Group 2003.

An estimated 75% of hospital admissions for asthma are avoidable and as many as 90% of the deaths from asthma are preventable.

Unfortunately, there is no cure for asthma. However, there are many effective treatments which, if used properly under guidance from your doctor or asthma nurse, should help you or your child to live normally and you should still be able to enjoy a healthy and active life. In other words, the goals of asthma treatment are to control your asthma.

What are the treatments available and are they safe?

The most effective way of taking your asthma treatment is through the use of an inhaler device, where the medicine is inhaled from your mouth into your airways. As the drug is going directly to your lungs, this means that you will need only a trace of the drug compared to if you were taking it in tablet or medicine form. The advantage of taking your asthma medication this way, is that very little of the medicine is absorbed into the rest of your body. It mostly reaches the target – your lungs.

The medicine that you need to control your asthma symptoms can be found in a variety of inhalers, which can often be confusing. It is essential that you are happy with your particular device and that you feel confident in using it. Your doctor or nurse will be able to advise you on which inhaler suits your particular needs. You can read about the different types of inhalers and devices in more detail in chapter 5.

As mentioned in chapter 1, the main groups of inhalers are relievers, preventers, protectors and combination therapy. Tablet medication is sometimes used in combination with your normal inhalers.

Short-acting bronchodilator therapy (Reliever therapy)

Everyone who has asthma should have one of these inhalers. This group of drugs can be used as soon as you feel breathless, have a wheeze, a tight chest or cough. These would be the symptoms that you would normally associate with asthma. The reliever immediately relaxes the smooth muscle fibres that line the outside of your main breathing tubes, the bronchus and bronchioles. These tubes start to constrict and twitch when they have been aggravated by a trigger, giving symptoms of a tight chest, a wheeze, shortness of breath or spasm. The reliever is used at step one of the National Asthma Guidelines (NAG - see Appendix A). Relievers offer quick release from your symptoms by opening your airways, allowing you to breathe more easily. However, they only work for around four hours at a time. As the relievers are essential at relieving asthma attacks, you should always have your reliever inhaler nearby as you never know when you might need it.

The two main relievers are known as Salbutamol and Terbutaline, although you may be more familiar with their varying brand names, depending on which company make them. Reliever inhalers are normally blue, but not always.

Children under the age of one may need a different kind of reliever more suited to their immature lungs. This drug is called Ipatropium Bromide and is classed as an 'anticholinergic' which works by also reducing spasm in the airways.

Reliever inhalers do have some harmless side effects that can be worrying. These side effects include a slight tremor or mild palpitations. If, for whatever reason, you need to use your reliever more than four times a week on a regular basis, or begin to wake at night due to your asthma symptoms, you will need to see your nurse or doctor, where they are likely offer you a preventer inhaler.

Inhaled corticosteroid therapy (Preventer therapy)

These inhalers contain low dose corticosteroids, which control the swelling and inflammation within your airways. This medication offers protection by stopping the tubes from being so sensitive to triggers and reduces the risks of severe asthma attacks. While relievers work straight away, preventers work over a space of time, often taking one to two weeks before becoming effective. This is why you would never use a preventer to treat an attack.

Inhaled steroids are introduced at step two of the National Asthma Guidelines. They are used in very small doses and as they are inhaled directly into your airways, again, none is absorbed into the rest of your body. They are a very safe and effective treatment. If your child requires preventer inhalers, then their growth will be carefully monitored.

The main generic names for preventer inhalers are, Beclometasone, Budesonide, Fluticasone, Ciclesonide, and Mometasone. They also have a number of branded names.

Relievers offer quick release from your symptoms by opening your airways, allowing you to breathe more easily.

Preventers are usually taken morning and night so you will not need to take them at school or at work. Once your asthma becomes well controlled, it is important to continue on your recommended dose of preventer medicine to keep your airways free from inflammation.

Your nurse or doctor will want to review you regularly as it can take some time to get the preventer dose right for your particular needs. Your health professional will be aiming to control your symptoms so effectively that you hardly need to rely on your reliever. This will mean that you have 'well-controlled asthma'. Once you gain control, continue using your preventer, remembering to take your reliever any time you develop symptoms. You will not be left on preventer medicine indefinitely. Your asthma symptoms can lay dormant for a while, so if you have been symptom free for about three months, under supervision of your nurse or doctor, you could reduce your inhaled preventer and monitor your symptoms.

Some common side effects of inhaled corticosteroids can include a dry mouth, a hoarse voice and thrush in your mouth. If you have any of these side effects, discuss them with your nurse or doctor. A simple switch to an inhaler device can reduce or alleviate these unwanted side effects. Also, side effects can be minimised by gargling and spitting out after using your inhaler or brushing your teeth afterwards. Using a spacer with your inhaler will help and these will be discussed in more detail in chapter five.

Long-acting bronchodilator therapy (Protector therapy)

The medicine in these inhalers works in a similar way to relievers by relaxing the smooth muscle fibres which open up your airways. Interestingly, they work for twelve hours at a time, so if taken in the morning and then again at night, they should offer protection throughout the day and night. Their generic names are Serevent, Oxis and Formoterol.

Common mild side effects of these inhalers include headache, sore throat and hoarseness. If you are concerned about any side effects, please discuss these with your doctor or nurse.

Long-acting bronchodilators are added in at step three of the National Asthma Guidelines (see Appendix A). They should only be used if you are already on an inhaled corticosteroid. These two medicines can be used in combination in one inhaler device which is discussed below.

Research has shown that by combining the drugs in one inhaler, there is a much better response to treatment.

Combination inhaler therapy

These inhalers are a combination of a low dose inhaled steroid mixed with a long-acting bronchodilator and they can be used for both adults and children. These are used at step three of the National Asthma Guidelines, when regular inhaled corticosteroids have not managed to help you gain good control. These inhalers work very well by relaxing the smooth muscle fibres in your airways as well as reducing the inflammation and mucus production. Where inhaled steroids work slowly over time, the combined inhalers work quickly. Usually improvement occurs within a few days. You can still use your normal reliever inhaler while you are waiting for your combination therapy to work fully.

The combination therapy can also be used separately, i.e. a separate long-acting bronchodilator and separate inhaled corticosteroid. Interestingly, research has shown that by combining the drugs in one inhaler, there is a much better response to treatment. Also, it means that they are easier to use as there are less inhalers to get used to.

The combination inhalers also come in differing colours and shapes. Devices will be covered in detail in chapter 5.

Leukotriene receptor antagonists

These are tablets that are taken at night, usually at step four of the NAG guidelines (see Appendix A), in mild to moderate asthma symptoms where a combination therapy inhaler is still not helping you to gain effective control. These tablets are taken as well as your combination therapy. They are particularly effective if you suffer with exercise-induced symptoms or have allergy-induced asthma symptoms. Leukotriene receptor antagonists (Singulair) are especially useful in children who are poorly controlled.

They work by reducing inflammation in a differing way to inhaled corticosteroids. They block one of the chemicals that is released when you come into contact with one of your triggers. Interestingly, these tablets also offer relief from hay fever. It can take up to a month to notice a full effect, so after four to six weeks, if you do not feel any benefit, then your doctor or nurse may suggest you stop.

Leukotriene receptor antagonists are taken once a day and are normally well tolerated. The more commonly reported side effects are stomach upsets, abdominal pain, headache and thirst. If you are worried about any side effects of the medications, you should make an appointment to discuss this with your doctor or asthma nurse. Often, side effects settle down quickly as your body gets used to your treatment.

Steroid tablets

A course of prednisolone tablets are used when someone is severely affected by their asthma. This is also known as rescue therapy. They are added to your usual asthma medication and are taken first thing in the morning. They are given as a short course, not usually more than one week and they quickly reverse the severe symptoms and help you to gain quick control. Although steroid tablets are given in high doses, they are given for a very short space of time and are perfectly safe when prescribed by a medical practitioner. Steroid tablets act by reducing the inflammation in your airways very quickly and effectively. This effect begins about eight hours after first starting the treatment. Very occasionally, someone with asthma may need to take daily oral prednisolone long-term, but this is unusual.

Theophylline tablets

This form of tablet medication is rarely used nowadays. It works by relaxing the muscles that surround the airways. Taking this twice-daily medicine also involves having regular blood tests. This type of medication is used sometimes in adults but normally they would be under strict supervision at an outpatient clinic at their local hospital.

Bronchodilator medicine

In some very small children, a bronchodilator in the form of a syrup can be given instead of using an inhaler. Some children find it very distressing using an inhaler with a spacer. For this reason, a syrup would be appropriate but it is important to remember that the syrup medicine can take a while to become effective whereby the bronchodilator inhaled medicine becomes effective immediately. It is always worth persevering with a small child in using an inhaler.

Compliance issues

It is well known that people often do not take their medications as prescribed by their doctors and asthmatic patients are no exception. One third of asthmatics stop their preventer inhalers as soon as they feel better. This premature withdrawal of the very effective anti-inflammatory effects of the inhaled steroids can, in some cases, be the causative factor in chronic (long-term) persistent asthma and acute (sudden) flare-ups.

Compliance problems can sometime be due to poor inhaler technique, fear of side effects, low expectations, lack of confidence in the treatment, or the device being used. Many parents express concerns about the long-term side effects of inhaled corticosteroids. They particularly have concerns about growth retardation in their children. This is one of the more common reasons why parents are reluctant for their children to use preventer inhalers. The truth is that used properly, with regular review, these anti-inflammatory inhalers are very safe and effective. They

It is well known that people often do not take their medications as prescribed by their doctors and asthmatic patients are no exception. One third of asthmatics stop their preventer inhalers as soon as they feel better.

are only used if necessary and your doctor or nurse will be keen to reduce the dose if your child's asthma symptoms are very well controlled. Your child's height will be measured at each consultation also.

Veena Rao et al (2008) looked at the effects of growth on children treated with inhaled and topical steroids for conditions such as asthma and eczema. They found that there was no difference in growth rates between patients receiving long-term steroid therapy and comparable patients with long-term illness who were not receiving steroids.

All of these problems can be easily addressed with your practice nurse or doctor, who will be only too happy to help you and relieve any anxieties that you may have.

Summing Up

- Always remember to have your reliever inhaler handy. You never know when an attack can occur.

- The goal of asthma treatment is to help control your asthma, in order that you can live a healthy, active life, free of symptoms. When your asthma is troublesome, your asthma treatment may need to be adjusted to gain quick control.

- Asthma inhalers are very safe with a small risk of side effects. As the drugs are being inhaled directly into your lungs, tiny doses will offer very effective treatment. Due to this, there is little absorption into the rest of your body.

- The inhaled drug groups are relievers, preventer, protectors and combination therapy.

- Other therapies can be taken by mouth and include anti-leukotrienes, theophylline and oral steroids.

- Oral steroids are used to treat sudden, worsening episodes of asthma called exacerbations which are given for a very short time to offer quick control of your symptoms.

- One of the most common causes of chronic asthma is due to compliance issues. If you have any concerns regarding your regular treatment, take a trip to see your practice nurse or doctor for advice. Remember to take your inhalers with you so that they can check your technique.

Types of Inhalers and Devices

As mentioned previously, most asthma treatment is given through an inhaler. There are many benefits in having your treatment this way. Firstly, the medicine travels directly to your airways as you only need a very small dose of the drug. Secondly, the drug will not enter your body as a whole which is what happens when you take your medicine by mouth.

'For many years, inhalation has been the preferred mode of administration of drugs for asthma, because this route offers several advantages. The drug is delivered directly to the affected organ, without undergoing systemic absorption, thus permitting a lower dose of medication to be used, reducing the potential for adverse side effects.'

Mark Levy, Linda Pearce. *Asthma*, Mosby, 2004.

There are many different types of devices so, for this reason, this chapter concentrates on the more popular devices currently used.

There are four main types of inhaled drug delivery system:

- Aerosol inhalers (pressurised metered dose inhalers).
- Powder inhalers (breath actuated inhalers).
- Inhalers with spacer devices.
- Nebulisers.

Your nurse or doctor will discuss and consider with you which inhaler device best suits your needs. If you are not able to use your inhaler correctly, you will not get enough of the drug into your lungs and this may result in your asthma becoming more of a problem for you.

Also, the clinician has to take into account the cost of your inhalers. This doesn't mean that you will be offered sub-standard treatment. It is the duty of any prescriber to consider the ongoing costs of all medications to the NHS. As there are so many treatments for asthma, you will be offered a treatment that is suited to your needs, safe and cost-effective.

Metered dose inhalers (MDI)

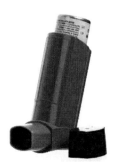

The metered dose aerosol inhalers are the most popular types of device. This is because they are often the cheapest with the greatest effect, especially if used with a spacer device. They have been in use for over forty years and are a very effective delivery system.

All of the differing drug treatments for asthma can be given through an MDI. They contain an inactive pressurised gas that propels a dose of drug with each puff. All of the inhaled drug groups can be given in this form.

How do I use my inhaler?

1 Sit in an upright position, remove the protective cap and shake your inhaler.

2 Breathe out fully, then hold the inhaler upright and place the mouthpiece into your mouth between your teeth, remembering to close your lips around it.

3 To release a dose of medicine, press the top of the canister and at the same time, breathe in deeply, then count slowly to ten or for as long as is comfortable.

4 If you need to take a second dose, wait for at least a minute before repeating from step 1.

5 Always remember to shake your device before using. If you do not wait at least a minute before using it again, the second dose will be gas and not a combination of drug and gas.

6 Replace the mouthpiece cover when finished.

● Remember to read the patient information leaflet that is supplied with your inhaler.

● Always remember to check the expiry date for your inhaler. Never use it if it has expired.

● Make sure that you order the prescriptions for your inhalers from your surgery before they run out.

● Remember to return all unused and empty inhalers to your pharmacy.

Some people find it difficult with the co-ordination that is required when using this inhaler. This is another reason why you should always take your inhaler with you when you have an appointment with your doctor or nurse. They will be able to check your technique.

Unfortunately, these inhalers often do not have a dose counter. This makes it difficult to decide if your inhaler is still active. The problem being that it runs out of drug long before the gas runs out. You will not be able to tell as you will still get the activation of the inhaler and it will taste the same. (See chapter 8 to find out how to check your inhaler.)

How do I care for my MDI?

- Do not wash the plastic device. The mouthpiece can be easily cleaned using an alcohol wipe.

- Store in a dry place and never above 30°C.

- If the canister becomes very cold, warm it up between your hands before using and push back into the plastic device.

Turbohalers

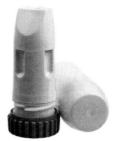

These inhalers are breath-actuated, dry powder inhalers and are very easy to use, especially for children. They also have a dose counter on the side and the last twenty doses appear in red. Also, the base locks when the device is empty.

Although easy to use and a very effective drug delivery system, these inhalers are more costly and are becoming less popular.

Relievers, preventers, protectors and combination drugs can all be given through a Turbohaler.

How do I use my Turbohaler?

1 Sitting in an upright position, unscrew the cover and lift it off.

2 Hold your inhaler upright with the coloured grip at the bottom.

3 To activate and load your Turbohaler, turn the coloured grip as far as it will go in one direction and then turn it in the opposite direction. You should then hear a 'click' sound. This means that your inhaler is ready to use.

4 Breathe out gently and then bring your inhaler to your mouth and place the mouthpiece between your teeth, then close your lips around the mouthpiece.

5 Breathe in as deeply and as hard as you can through your mouth. Do not bite the mouthpiece.

6 Remove the Turbohaler from your mouth but remember to hold your breath for about ten seconds or for as long as is comfortable.

7 If you need to take a second dose then repeat steps two to six.

You may wish to rinse your mouth out and spit out. This helps reduce any unwanted side effects. When you have finished, always remember to replace the protective cover.

Remember that you will probably not taste anything when using this inhaler, but if you have used it correctly, you can be sure that you have had a dose.

How do I care for my Turbohaler?

- To clean your inhaler, all you need to do is to wipe the mouthpiece once a week with a dry tissue.

- Do not clean it with water or any liquids.

- Store your inhaler in a dry place and never above 30°C.

Accuhaler inhaler

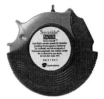

This type of inhaler is a breath-actuated, dry powder inhaler. It is used for relievers, preventers, protectors and combination therapy. It is very easy to use and so is often used for children. The Accuhaler does have a dose counter and when you are on your final five doses, the counter turns red.

How do I use my Accuhaler?

1 To open your Accuhaler, hold the outer case in one hand and place the thumb of your other hand on the thumb grip. Push your thumb away from you and feel the inhaler slide open. If you push it as far as it will go, you will hear a click sound.

2 Hold the inhaler so that the mouthpiece is facing your mouth, then slide the lever away from you again, until you hear another click. Your inhaler is now ready to use.

3 Breathe out for as long as you can and then bring the mouthpiece towards you, placing it between your lips. Remember to close your lips around the mouthpiece to make a seal.

4 Breathe in steadily and deeply and then take it out of your mouth, remembering to hold your breath for about ten seconds or for as long as is comfortable.

5 Now close your inhaler by sliding the thumb grip back towards you until you hear a click. The lever will automatically return to its resting position.

6 If you need to take a second dose then repeat from step one.

How do I care for my Accuhaler?

- To clean your Accuhaler, wipe the mouthpiece with a dry tissue and do not allow it to get wet.

- Store in a cool dry place, never above 30°C.

Autohalers

 Again, all of the drug groups can be given effectively through this type of inhaler. It is also a breath-actuated, aerosol CFC-free inhaler which has an audible 'click' when activated. One drawback is that there is no dose counter.

How do I use my Autohaler?

1 Remove the mouthpiece cover by pushing down on the lip of the device at the back of the cover.

2 Shake the inhaler and then push the grey leaver upwards. This primes the inhaler and it is now ready to use.

3 Breathe out and then close your lips around the mouthpiece tightly. There are ventilation holes underneath the device so make sure your hand does not block these.

4 Breathe in slowly and deeply and continue to inhale after the device has fired when you will hear a click sound.

5 Hold your breath for as long as you can, although try for at least ten seconds.

6 If you need to take a second dose, push the grey lever down and repeat from step 2. You should wait about a minute before taking a second dose.

How do I care for my Autohaler?

- When you use this inhaler for the first time, you should fire off two doses to prime it for use. This is done by pushing forward the white lever on the underside of the inhaler.

- Do not allow your inhaler to get wet. The mouthpiece can be cleaned with an alcohol wipe.

- Store in a cool, dry place.

Easi-Breathe inhalers

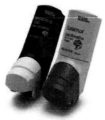

This inhaler is an aerosol breath-actuated CFC-free device. It has an audible sound when it fires, and sounds like a gentle puff. Unfortunately, there is no dose counter either. The Easi-Breathe device comes with an optimiser which acts like a small spacer, slowing down the drug particles and allowing better drug deposition into the lungs.

How do I use my Easi-Breathe inhaler?

1 First, shake your inhaler.

2 Open the cap which is attached to the underside by a hinge and covers the mouthpiece. Opening the cap primes the device.

3 Now breathe out slowly.

4 Ensuring that your hand doesn't obstruct the air holes on the top of the device, place the mouthpiece firmly between your teeth and place your lips around with a tight seal. Breathe in slowly and deeply through the mouthpiece. You will hear the dose being released by an audible puffing sound. Continue to breathe in slowly and then hold your breath for as long is comfortable, usually about ten seconds.

5 Breathe out slowly and then close the cap whilst holding the inhaler upright.

6 If you need to take another puff, wait about a minute before repeating from step 1.

How do I care for my Easi-Breathe inhaler?

- Clean your inhaler with a clean, dry cloth. It should be stored in a cool, dry place.

- Do not allow it to get wet.

Spacers/aerochambers

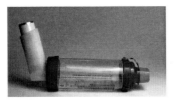

There are a number of differing types of spacers and to describe all of these would be beyond the scope of this book. Generally speaking, spacers slow down the delivery of the drug which in turn reduces side effects of the inhaled medication, particularly the more common unwanted effects of a dry mouth or sore throat. Spacers also help to improve drug deposition. They are very useful and particularly good for use with small children and the elderly. Spacers are usually only prescribed with pressurised MDIs.

Spacers have another added benefit. With the best inhaler technique possible, you will only get about 10-15% of your drug delivered to your lungs by using your inhaler alone. The remaining drug hits the back of the throat and is swallowed and then excreted through your kidneys and bowel. This applies to all of the inhalers that are used without a spacer.

Interestingly, when your MDI is used through a spacer, you will get 90% of the drug delivered into your lung tissue, therefore a more effective result in terms of symptom control. Spacers are becoming more popular. Smaller ones are now available and they have the added advantage of being more transportable, carried easily in handbags or school bags. The older, bigger spacers were cumbersome to carry and for that reason, people didn't seem to like to use them.

Also, in an emergency situation, a Ventolin MDI (reliever) used through a spacer is a very effective way to treat an exacerbation while you are waiting for an ambulance or on the way to hospital. Spacers are just as good at delivering your medicine compared to nebulisers.

The spacer is very simple to use. The MDI fits securely into one end and you will find a mouthpiece at the other. The chamber holds the drug to be inhaled and near the mouthpiece there is a valve that allows your exhaled breath to escape but not the drug. A face mask can be fitted for anyone who cannot make a seal, for example children or the elderly.

When your MDI is used through a spacer, you will get 90% of the drug delivered into your lung tissue, therefore a more effective result in terms of symptom control.

How do I use my spacer?

1 Take one puff at a time.

2 Once the MDI inhaler is slotted into place, shake the whole device before activating it.

3 Place the mouthpiece in your mouth, press the canister and inhale deeply and slowly, holding your breath slightly and then breathing out slowly and again, breathing in deeply and holding. In other words, take two deep breaths per activation. If you need to take another dose, shake the whole device and repeat.

How do I care for my spacer?

- Your spacer should be cleaned monthly, by agitating it in warm soapy water and then rinsing and leaving to drip dry.

- Do not dry with a paper towel as this will create static charge and the drug will stick to the inside of the chamber, therefore less drug will be inhaled.

Nebulisers

Some people purchase their own nebulisers off the Internet and I have known some even buy them at car boot sales. This has to be discouraged and is dangerous.

The nebuliser is a machine which uses compressed air that flows through tubing, which is fixed to a mask or mouthpiece. The nebuliser turns your liquid asthma medicine into a mist, which you inhale. Also, the nebuliser can be used with oxygen. A nebuliser is mainly used in hospital, to treat a sudden asthma attack (acute exacerbation) but some people use nebulisers at home. The nurse may use one from time to time when an asthmatic attends the surgery whist having an acute attack. People with poor manual dexterity and those with severe learning disabilities may also benefit from using a nebuliser.

Some people purchase their own nebulisers off the Internet and I have known some even buy them at car boot sales. This has to be discouraged and is dangerous. The nebulisers that are used in hospitals and GPs surgeries are checked and maintained regularly to ensure that they are working properly. Also, regarding cross-infection issues, the nebuliser kits, which comprise of masks and tubing, should only be used by one person and should be replaced regularly.

If you have your own nebuliser which has been given to you by your doctor or an outpatients' clinic, it is important that you have it serviced regularly and that it is kept in good working order. Your regular supplier should give you advice regarding this.

How do I use my nebuliser?

Again, as there are many types of nebulisers, describing each one is beyond the scope of this book. Detailed instructions will come with the nebuliser and you can ask your provider for any help that you need in terms of using and cleaning your nebuliser and ordering face masks, tubing and mouthpieces.

Peak flow meters

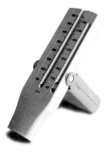

As shown, a peak flow meter is a small, plastic, inexpensive, portable, hand-held device which helps you to measure how much air your lungs can blow out in one quick blow. Your peak flow readings will vary depending on your age, height and gender. Your doctor or nurse will be able to predict what your usual peak flow readings should be using a prediction chart using these indicators. When your asthma is troublesome, this causes airflow obstruction and your peak flow readings will drop in response to this.

Depending on how far the levels drop from your normal best blow, your nurse or doctor will be able to show you what to do next when your asthma symptoms are troublesome. Using a peak flow meter in managing your asthma will be discussed in more detail in chapter 7.

How do I use my peak flow meter?

1 Sit or stand up straight and remove any gum or food from your mouth.

2 Check the cursor or arrow is on zero.

3 Take a deep breath and place the peak flow mouthpiece in your mouth with your lips tightly closed, keeping your tongue away from the mouthpiece. Hold the meter level and blow as hard and as fast as you can.

4 The force of the air moves the cursor up the number scale. Make sure you write the number down.

5 Return the cursor to zero and repeat the blow a second and third time. If the three numbers are very near to each other, this means that you have blown correctly.

6 Record the highest of the three recordings in your peak flow chart. If you do not have one, can ask your doctor or nurse for a chart.

Summing Up

- Asthma treatment is normally delivered by inhalation, more commonly through an inhaler, but sometimes through a spacer and less commonly, through a nebuliser.

- Your nurse or doctor will work in partnership with you in deciding which inhaler device suits your needs and abilities.

- Metered dose inhalers (MDIs) are the most popular aerosol device.

- Turbohalers, Accuhalers, Easi-Breathe inhalers and Autohalers are all breath-actuated inhalers.

- Spacers are generally used with MDIs and they deliver the drug to the lung tissue more efficiently and more effectively. They also help reduce the risk of any unwanted side effects.

- Nebulisers are used mostly in hospital during an asthma exacerbation or for home use in very poorly people.

Smoking and Asthma

Tobacco smoke is known to be an irritant. In asthma, it doesn't necessarily trigger an allergic reaction, but it irritates airways that are already inflamed and irritated. This in turn will worsen asthma and trigger your asthma symptoms. Sometimes it can cause a severe asthma attack which is both dangerous and very frightening.

Some studies show that teenagers who smoke more than 300 cigarettes per year are four times more likely to develop asthma as a result.

The National Heart, Lung and Blood Institute go so far as to say that asthmatics should never smoke or be exposed to passive tobacco smoke.

As a parent or teacher, it is so important to warn older children and teenagers about the harmful effects of cigarette smoking.

Some studies show that teenagers who smoke more than 300 cigarettes per year are four times more likely to develop asthma as a result.

'Tobacco smoke can aggravate asthma symptoms or trigger an attack. According to an Asthma UK survey, tobacco smoke is a trigger for more than 80% of people with asthma.'

Asthma UK – *People with asthma at work*.

What are the effects of smoking on asthma?

Exposure to tobacco smoke is one of the most destructive irritants regarding your asthma, made worse if it is in an indoor environment. Also, smoking can permanently damage your airways, increase your chance of having an asthma attack and reduce the effectiveness of your inhalers. It can also lead to irreversible airways disease, commonly called chronic obstructive pulmonary disease, which includes lung conditions such as emphysema and bronchiectasis. Smoking also increases the risk of persistent asthma in teenagers who smoke.

Does smoking in pregnancy increase the risk of a baby developing asthma?

Unfortunately, if you smoke during pregnancy, you put your baby at a higher risk of developing asthma, being born prematurely, having a low birth weight and increasing your risk of having a miscarriage. Also smoking in pregnancy could make your asthma worse.

You can access help on the NHS Pregnancy Smoking Helpline on 0800 169 9 169. Alternatively, you can access their help on www.givingupsmoking.co.uk.

This has been set up with trained advisors who can provide information and help you to stop. More information can be found in the help list section at the back of this book.

How does passive smoking affect us?

- Passive smoking relates to when we inhale second-hand smoke from other people's cigarettes and cigars. This second-hand smoke exposes all of us to health risks, including asthma.

- Where a child is exposed to second-hand smoke, this will increase their chance of developing asthma five-fold and they are twice as likely to have chest infections.

- Where babies are exposed, this can increase the risk of cot death.

- Where adults are exposed to second-hand smoke, their risk of developing asthma doubles.

- Second-hand smoke can linger for two and a half hours even if the window is open.

- Passive smoking has been shown to reduce your lung function, increase your need for your asthma medicine and increase your need for time off work or school due to your symptoms.

- Research shows that smoking around children is the main cause of 35,000 preventable hospital and GP visits per year.

Where a child is exposed to second-hand smoke, this will increase their chance of developing asthma five-fold and they are twice as likely to have chest infections.

The *Take 7 Steps Out* government campaign is a recent drive designed at promoting the importance of reducing the effects of passive smoking by, not only going outside to smoke, but to take seven steps once you get outside, therefore reducing the immediate and life-long impact of second-hand smoke. It is claimed that these simple strategies will reduce the effect of passive smoking on cot deaths, middle ear infections and asthma attacks.

More reasons to stop smoking

Nicotine, one of the many substances found in cigarettes, is a highly addictive drug. Stopping smoking can be difficult but with the right help and information it is entirely possible. Many people stop smoking every day in the UK.

Stopping smoking is the single most positive step to improving your health and increasing your chances of living a longer life. Quitting smoking will also reduce your risk of developing chronic diseases such as asthma, chronic obstructive airways disease, emphysema, heart disease, cancer of the lung and throat, hypertension; the list goes on!

It is important to remember that trying to stop smoking is an ongoing process. Many people who quit have tried a number of times before they are successful. This is normal, so don't beat yourself up if you don't manage to stop. Just pick yourself up again when you feel motivated and have another go. Keep on trying and you will give up one day.

- After 20 minutes of stopping, your blood pressure and pulse will return to normal.

- After 8 hours of stopping, your chance of having a heart attack is already falling.

- After 24 hours, you will start to clear mucus and debris from your lungs.

- After 48 hours, nicotine has completely left your body. Your sense of taste and smell is improving.

- After 72 hours, your lungs are functioning more normally.

- After 3-9 months, your lung function improves by 10%.

- After 5 years, you have reduced your risk of having a heart attack by half.

- After 10 years, you have reduced your chance of getting lung cancer by 50%.

Preparing to stop

Massive steps were taken towards a smoke-free future in 2007, when a ban on smoking in enclosed public areas and workplaces became law. Infact, I have come into contact with many ex-smokers who say that this ban really helped them to stop. Prior to the ban and in the comfort of a cosy pub, there was nothing to prevent a friend from offering them a cigarette. After a few drinks had weakened their resolve, it could be difficult to say no.

However, since the ban, and through not being in contact with cigarette smoke, 'quitters' are much less likely to be tempted. Also, it now seems to be socially acceptable for those trying to quit to sit inside, whilst their smoking friends nip out for a quick cigarette.

You have a much better chance of giving up if you prepare to quit in advance. Why not try and keep a diary of the times when you smoke? This will help you identify the difficult times in your day which will challenge you. If you know when your usual times are for smoking, you may be able to introduce changes to help reduce the trigger to smoke.

Perhaps if you always smoke at the breakfast table while drinking a cup of coffee and reading the paper,

Change things by drinking tea and watching telly instead. This reduces your psychological triggers. Also, make a list of all the reasons why you want to give up smoking and pin this to key places in your home.

After 10 years, you have reduced your chance of getting lung cancer by 50%.

Put all your smoking money in a jar and watch it grow. Treat yourself to something nice as a reward for stopping smoking. This could be a new handbag, sports equipment or booking a long weekend away or even a holiday. Perhaps plan to have driving lessons with your smoking money. What a great reward to enjoy!

If a friend offers you a cigarette, don't reply by saying, 'No thanks, I'm trying to give up!'. Make a much more positive declaration by saying, 'No thanks. I don't smoke!'

This way you will make more of a positive impact, and who knows, your friend may try and give up too! Once you've decided on a quit date, throw all your ashtrays and lighters away. Throw any unused cigarettes away.

Accessing help

Did you know that you are four times more likely to stop smoking if you are given support and nicotine replacement therapy (NRT) than if you go it alone using just willpower.

You can access help to stop smoking from many sources. Most GP surgeries have at least one health professional trained in helping people to quit. They will also be fully aware of the currently available smoking cessation therapies that can aid your success in quitting. Why don't you ring and ask reception what services they provide.

Research shows that if you set a quit date and prepare for this, you will have a much better chance of success. Your doctor or nurse will try and help you set a quit date. Also, they can arrange for you to attend your local specialist cessation services. You may be offered one-to-one help, or group therapy.

Some smokers find alternative therapies such as acupuncture, herbal medicines, meditation or hypnosis to be beneficial.

You can also access help to quit by visiting www.nhs.uk/smokefree.

Here you will be able to arrange face-to-face smoking cessation help with an advisor. You can also request one-to-one or group work therapy. Alternatively, many chemists and pharmacists have specialist skills in supporting those trying to quit. They often run 'stop smoking programmes' which are affordable and very supportive.

> **Research shows that if you set a quit date and prepare for this, you will have a much better chance of success.**

Nicotine replacement therapy and other treatments explained

When you stop smoking, your body is trying to cope with the effects of nicotine withdrawal, while your mind will try to deal with psychological dependence.

The term 'psychological dependence' relates to the habit of smoking and the triggers in the day when it is time to smoke, for example you might always have a cigarette at breakfast whilst reading the morning paper. The habit trigger may be kicking in without you experiencing a physical withdrawal trigger to smoke.

The term 'physical dependence' relates to your body's nicotine dependence and stopping smoking makes coping with nicotine withdrawal difficult. Some people have worse withdrawal symptoms than others. Giving up can be made easier with a number of modern therapies, all of which help reduce physical and sometimes psychological withdrawal from cigarettes.

Currently, there are two smoking cessation treatment options available on the NHS. They are nicotine replacement therapy, which comes in many forms and tablet medication called Champix and Zyban. Remember, you can access these treatments through a stop smoking clinic at your GP surgery. Alternatively, you can contact the NHS Smoking Helpline (see help list for details).

Nicotine replacement therapy (NRT)

This treatment comes in the form of patches, gum, lozenges, micro tabs, nasal spray and an inhalator and is normally used for a treatment period of ten to twelve weeks. However, it can be used for longer. NRT works by reducing the physical withdrawal associated with stopping smoking and can be used in pregnancy and during breastfeeding.

Zyban

This oral medication has an effect of inhibiting the reuptake of chemicals noradrenalin and dopamine, thereby reducing your cravings and withdrawal. The treatment is usually prescribed for seven to nine weeks. This treatment has to be prescribed with caution due to unpleasant side effects and it should not be used in anyone who has suffered with epilepsy, brain tumours, bulimia or anorexia, bipolar disorder, liver disease or anyone experiencing abrupt withdrawal from alcohol. Zyban cannot be used in pregnancy or during breastfeeding.

Champix

This treatment is a more popular smoking cessation therapy and is very effective. It works by binding to nicotine receptors in your brain to alleviate withdrawal symptoms. Champix also reduces the pleasurable effect of nicotine. Compared to Zyban, Champix appears to be safer in terms of its side effect profile, but it needs to be used with caution in those who have a past medical history of psychiatric conditions, including depression. Champix is used normally for a three-month period. Champix cannot be used in pregnancy or during breastfeeding.

Summing Up

- Tobacco smoke is a known irritant which worsens your asthma symptoms. This happens even if you inhale second-hand smoke.

- Smoking can permanently damage your airways, causing irreversible lung disease.

- Smoking in pregnancy increases your baby's risk of developing asthma as well as being born prematurely, of low birth weight or ending in miscarriage.

- You can access help to stop smoking from your local GP or nurse, your pharmacist or you can ring various sources as shown in the help list at the end of this book.

- Setting a quit date will help you to plan ahead. This will increase your chances of quitting successfully.

- Current popular treatments to help you quit successfully are nicotine replacement therapy and anti-smoking tablets such as Zyban and Champix.

How to Recognise and Manage an Attack

What are the reasons for sudden attacks?

Unfortunately, despite being careful, taking your inhalers and avoiding your triggers, you may still suffer from an attack or exacerbation. As mentioned previously, asthma can be triggered as a result of the simple cold or flu virus and other respiratory infections such as rhinovirus. Boys seem to have a higher risk of exacerbation in childhood and women more at risk in adulthood. A direct link has been identified between two infections named chlamydophila pneumoniae and mycoplasma pneumoniae in causing severe sudden asthma exacerbations. The importance of immunisation against influenza and pneumonia will be discussed more fully in chapter 8.

Surprisingly, the pollen season often starts at the end of February, where the trees begin to shed their pollen. Often, during the spring and early summer, asthma can become very unstable.

Exacerbations in pregnancy usually occur in the late second trimester and it has been found the major triggers for this are as a result of viral infections and through poor compliance in taking inhaled corticosteroids preventer therapy. If a woman has an exacerbation during pregnancy, there is an increased risk of the baby being born of low birth weight. For this reason, it is crucial that asthma is well managed during pregnancy.

Some pregnant mothers worry about the long-term effects on the baby's development if the mother needs to use preventer steroid therapy. There is minimal risk. It is far more risky for a baby if the mother's asthma is poorly controlled during pregnancy.

Interestingly, unpredictable, bizarre weather appears to be an alarming trigger for asthma. In the spring of 2007, due to the very warm, dry weather, many more than usual patients experienced severe, sudden symptoms when they were normally well controlled.

Thunderstorm asthma is a new phenomenon, not normally associated with respiratory disease. However, its effects are extremely alarming. On the evening of 23rd of June 2005, warnings of severe thunderstorms were issued from the Met Office. The following evening, hospital accident and emergency departments in the northwest of London were swamped with people attending with sudden asthma exacerbations. The number of asthmatics requiring emergency treatment

Thunderstorm asthma is a new phenomenon. On the evening of 23rd of June 2005, warnings of severe thunderstorms were issued from the Met Office. The following evening, hospital accident and emergency departments in the northwest of London were swamped with people attending with sudden asthma exacerbations.

was eight times the normal rate. Many hospital departments ran out of the emergency nebuliser treatment that was required to quickly and effectively reverse their symptoms.

For those of you who may be allergic to aspirin, you may notice that certain foods can trigger exacerbations. These are foods that contain salicylate which can trigger a bad attack. These foods will be discussed more fully in chapter 10.

Also, if you're allergic to aspirin, you may also be allergic to non-steroidal anti-inflammatories such as ibuprofen, naproxen, diclofenac and meloxicam. These should be taken with extreme caution if you have asthma.

Asthma exacerbations are very frightening and, unfortunately, they can be fatal. It is important that you know how to recognise when an attack is looming and what to do in an emergency. If you think that you are having an attack, whatever time of day or night it is, never be afraid to call for an ambulance. Even if your symptoms settle, it is never a waste of time.

'If you notice your asthma symptoms are getting worse you should take your reliever inhaler.'

Breathing well – Asthma Advice – Chiesi LTD.

How can I tell when an attack may be on the way?

Often, before an attack, there are common signs that your asthma is poorly controlled and that an attack is looming. These signs are:

- Waking in the night coughing, wheezing or short of breath.

- Falling peak flow.

- Needing to use your reliever inhaler more than usual and its effect not lasting as long.

- Waking earlier than normal and needing to use your reliever inhaler.

The above are all signs that you or your child's asthma is poorly controlled and you should make plans to see your doctor or asthma nurse as soon as possible.

You are having an asthma attack if:

- Your reliever inhaler does not relieve your symptoms.

- You are too breathless to talk, eat or sleep.

- Your symptoms of cough, wheeze, breathlessness or tight chest are out of control.

At the time of your asthma attack, try and do a peak flow reading. If your result is 50% or less of your usual result when you are well, this will confirm that you are having a severe attack. After having your reliever inhaler, recheck your peak flow. If it is still at 50% or less of your usual recording, you need to call an ambulance.

If a child is having an attack and they are under the age of eight, they will probably not be able to perform a peak flow reading.

Also, it is important to note the differences between the way in which small children and adults behave during an attack. A small child or infant may not appear distressed and may just appear quiet and relaxed during an attack. Do not be fooled. If a child or infant is stooping forward or dribbling or excessively yawning, then this is severe.

Now:

1 Take two puffs of your reliever inhaler which is usually blue.

2 Sit quietly and try to control your breathing.

3 If you do not feel any relief from your inhaler take another two puffs of your inhaler every two minutes up until ten puffs have been taken.

4 If you do not feel any improvement, call 999.

5 If you have to wait for an ambulance for a while, you can repeat step 3 again to ease your breathing.

If after step three you feel much better, it is important to still make an appointment at your surgery and see the doctor or your asthma nurse as soon as possible. The fact that you needed to take much more than your usual reliever inhaler tells you that your asthma is very out of control. Get seen as soon as you can.

If after step three you feel much better, it is important to still make an appointment at your surgery and see the doctor or your asthma nurse as soon as possible. The fact that you needed to take much more than your usual reliever inhaler tells you that your asthma is very out of control. Get seen as soon as you can.

If you are admitted to hospital to manage your symptoms, it is very important that you also book an appointment with your doctor or asthma nurse within 48 hours of being discharged from hospital. This is important, as you will need to be closely assessed.

If you are a school teacher, it is your responsibility to know who in your class has asthma. You also need to ensure that those children are able to get to their reliever inhalers as soon as they need it as any delay could prove very dangerous. If you are not sure, find out what your school policy is and ask about training or a refresher course if you feel that your skills need updating.

Also, make sure that the dinner ladies or helpers are aware of the needs of asthmatic children. My daughter, at the age of seven, asked during lunch break if she could go and get her inhaler. The dinner lady observing in the playground told her to wait until the end of break. You can imagine how worrying this was for me as a parent!

If you have a spacer device, remember that much more of the drug is able to be delivered to the lungs, so use this if you can during an attack. If your usual reliever inhaler fits into a spacer but you do not have a spacer with you, you can improvise by using a plastic drinking cup. Cut out a hole in the bottom, big enough to insert the mouthpiece of your inhaler and then place the lip of the cup over your mouth and nose and use as you would when using a spacer.

Who to call during an attack

As previously mentioned, if your usual reliever inhaler is not working and you fear that you are having an asthma attack as above, call 999, sit quietly and try to keep calm. Continue to use your reliever inhaler while you are waiting.

What is the difference between an asthma attack and a panic attack?

Anxiety and panic attacks are very unpleasant, common conditions. Often a sufferer is not aware of the cause of their anxiety. It does become complicated when a person with asthma starts to have a panic attack as the symptoms are very similar. It is important that you are able to tell the difference if you or another person or child is having breathing difficulties. The symptoms could be a result of either asthma or anxiety or both. Obviously, anxiety will play a part in an asthma attack as it is very frightening.

Sometimes anxiety alone can trigger an attack in those who are susceptible.

Fear of the condition alone can cause anxiety in asthmatics or anyone caring for them. Visiting your asthma nurse or doctor for regular check-ups can arm you with knowledge of your asthma and this will help reduce the anxiety around this condition.

Both conditions can cause shortness of breath, a tight chest, feeling anxious with palpitations and difficulty in speaking. However, the main differences between an asthma attack and a panic attack are as follows:

In asthma:

- You will have a wheeze or cough with a reduced peak expiratory flow rate.

In a panic attack:

- You will probably feel dizzy and lightheaded. You may have cramps. You will be 'over-breathing' or hyperventilating. If you feel tingling in your fingers or lips, then this is more likely to be a panic attack.

Sometimes anxiety alone can trigger an attack in those who are susceptible.

How do I control my panic symptoms?

There are a number of steps you can take to help control these symptoms. In a sudden attack, it helps to sit quietly and try and control your breathing. During a panic attack which results in over-breathing or hyperventilating, you take in too much oxygen which causes the tingling in your lips and fingers. This can be reduced by breathing in your own carbon dioxide and then your oxygen levels will fall to normal levels. This is easily accomplished by using a paper bag or large envelope. Scrunch it up so that there is a small opening at the end which you will use to seal around your mouth and continue to breathe in and out slowly, all the time keeping the opening of the bag or envelope fixed to your lips.

If you do not have a bag or envelope, try breathing out fully, holding your breath for as long as you can and when you can no longer do this, slowly breathe in but don't overfill your lungs. Again, slowly breathe out fully and hold your breath for as long as you can. This will calm your breathing and reduce your symptoms.

Yoga and Buteyko breathing exercises are useful. These techniques will be discussed more fully in chapter 10.

Try visiting your doctor and ask if you can be referred for cognitive behavioural therapy (CBT). This is an excellent treatment for all anxiety disorders. It is very effective with long-term results. Your doctor may also suggest some medication to help. This will be prescribed safely and you will be monitored in order to ensure that the treatment is working for you without any side effects. Your doctor may suggest a referral for a course of counselling or talking therapy.

You could visit your library where you will be able to find a large selection of books on meditation and relaxation therapies, including relaxation techniques. Also, a wide selection of DVDs are available. Some doctors' surgeries offer 'books on prescription' through the NHS services. These books can be lent to you through your local library services for eight weeks at a time. Enquire at your local library to see if they offer this excellent service.

Perhaps regular massage would be more appealing for you? If you live near a local college who teach massage, you may be able to get free or very much reduced cost massages as they are often looking for volunteers for their students to practise their skills on.

Any form of exercise is good for the mind and body. During exercise, we release the 'happy endorphins' which give you a natural 'high' and are great for helping reduce stress and anxiety. This can also be used as a great distraction technique. If you could incorporate it with learning a new skill, such as figure skating or tennis, not only will you be getting excellent exercise, you will also have a positive sense of achievement. This will increase your self-esteem and confidence also.

Summing Up

- Asthma attacks are caused by triggers. Common triggers include house dust mite, pollen, animal dander, perfumes and chemicals, as a result of a viral infection and sensitivity to some drugs, such as aspirin or non-steroidal anti-inflammatories.

- Signs of poorly controlled asthma include, night-time waking to use your inhaler, falling peak flow, needing to use your reliever inhaler more frequently, and early morning waking in order to use your reliever.

- You are having an asthma attack if your reliever is not reversing your symptoms, if you are too breathless to talk, eat or sleep, and your symptoms are out of control.

- During an attack, a spacer device can be used with your reliever to improve the effectiveness of the relieving medication.

- Asthma and panic symptoms can feel very similar. The main differences are that in panic, you may experience cramps, tingling fingers or lips, and over-breathing or hyperventilating.

- As a teacher, ensure that you are aware who the asthmatics are in your class and ensure that they can always get to their inhaler during class time and playtime.

8

Making the Most of Your Review

What is the role of my general practitioner?

For a number of years now, people with long-term conditions such as asthma, hypertension, heart disease, chronic obstructive pulmonary disease, kidney disease and diabetes have had most of their care delivered by practice nurses who attend training to enable them to provide excellent, up-to-date care and treatment. They can often be more up to date than the doctors.

If your condition seems very complicated and the nurse needs some advice, then the doctor acts as a point of contact to offer support and guidance. Often, the GPs will take a lead role in a long-term condition and will work together with the nurse during a specific clinic time, although this varies from surgery to surgery.

Most health concerns are dealt with at surgery level but where the outcome is not satisfactory, or the disease pathway is not expected, the doctor may refer you to hospital for a second opinion.

> For a number of years now, people with long-term conditions, such as asthma, have had most of their care delivered by practice nurses who attend training to enable them to provide excellent, up-to-date care and treatment.

What is the role of the asthma nurse?

The nurses within general practice attend updates and courses, providing them with information and education. This in turn, helps them to offer you an up-to-date and effective service to help you manage your long-term condition of asthma. Some surgeries may have more than one nurse offering this excellent service.

The role of the nurse is to:

- Keep an up-to-date register of all asthmatic patients.
- Provide information about this long-term condition to assist you to manage your condition more effectively.
- Teach you how to use your inhalers correctly, how to clean them and show you how to tell when they are empty.
- Help you to identify your personal triggers, so that, if at all possible, you may be able to avoid some of them.
- Operate a system where you will receive invites to attend your asthma review and contact you if you have not been able to attend.
- Effectively audit the service that they provide.

The nurses have many ways to identify who is having trouble with their asthma. Just by looking at how many reliever inhalers that you have requested over a period of time, can tell her how well or badly controlled your asthma is.

The aim of asthma care is, with a range of therapies available, to control your asthma so well that you hardly ever need to use your reliever inhaler. If you have mild asthma and you only rarely need to use your reliever inhaler, then congratulations, you are already deemed well controlled.

The nurses can only help you to achieve effective control if you attend the surgery for your review. The nurses can give you loads of information about your inhalers and leaflets that will support this information.

In cases of pollen trigger, your nurse will be able to help you identify the months or weeks of the year where you will be more at risk and she will show you how to take steps to reduce the effect of your triggers and how to control your asthma more effectively. For example, if you are always more troubled in March, due to tree pollen, then she may encourage you to 'step up' your treatment just beforehand, so that your triggers are less troublesome. If you need to use a reliever occasionally, then you would be put on an inhaled corticosteroids (preventer) a few weeks beforehand, to maintain control of your symptoms, and then you would be 'stepped down' to your usual treatment, once your trigger had subsided. This will be supported with a written individual action plan, tailored to your needs.

The aim of asthma management is:

- No daytime symptoms.
- No night-time waking due to asthma.
- No need for rescue medication.
- No exacerbations.
- No exercise limitations.
- Normal lung function.

In cases of pollen trigger, your nurse will be able to help you identify the months or weeks of the year where you will be more at risk and she will show you how to take steps to reduce the effect of your triggers and how to control your asthma more effectively.

What should I expect from my asthma review?

Your asthma review is very important. You will only learn to control your condition and learn how to identify when it is becoming out of control if you attend regularly for your reviews.

At this appointment the nurse will:

- Discuss your current day and night symptoms with you.
- Check your inhaler technique.
- Check your peak expiratory flow rate.
- Discuss your known triggers.
- Offer support and advice, backed up by leaflets.
- If you have a child with asthma then their height and weight should be measured regularly.

Many people make the mistake of only seeing the doctor or asthma nurse when their asthma is troubling them. If only they had attended more frequently. Through regular help and ongoing education, these people may have recognised earlier when their symptoms were out of control and would have been able to alter their treatment earlier.

During a review you should expect to be asked the following three questions:

Have you had difficulty sleeping because of your asthma symptoms (including cough)?

Have you had your usual asthma symptoms during the day (cough, wheeze, chest tightness or breathlessness)?

Has your asthma interfered with your usual activities (e.g. housework or work)?

Asthma UK – *Making the most of your Asthma Review*

Some people may record their peak flow reading at home, in an asthma diary, on a regular basis. If you have become more symptomatic, requiring a change in your regular treatment, then checking your peak flow at home is a great idea. Remember to always take your asthma diary, peak flow meter and inhalers to your appointment.

By having a regular review, your nurse or doctor will be able to help you to achieve much better control of your symptoms. This will also reduce your risks of exacerbations and time off work or school.

What is self-management planning?

With guidance from your nurse or doctor, you will learn the skills to manage your condition effectively. Through education and understanding your condition fully, you will then be more active in identifying independently, when your symptoms are becoming more of a problem. You will then have the confidence and knowledge to alter your treatment accordingly and will know when to seek help from your nurse.

Your nurse will help you identify what to do when you are bothered by your asthma and how to adjust your treatment. This will be supported by a personal written action plan. All of these activities are to encourage self-management planning.

Confidence and understanding your condition and varying treatments take a lot of time. You will never be expected to know it all.

Confidence and understanding your condition and varying treatments takes a lot of time. You will never be expected to know it all, and your nurse and doctor are there to help you at all times. If you are unable to grasp the concept of self-management, do not worry. It sometimes takes years to develop these skills and your nurse or doctor are there to help you at every step of the way.

Also, if you are unsure about your medication in any way, always ask your clinician. Everyone has a different level of understanding and a differing rate of learning. Your nurse and doctor know this. They will tailor your education about your condition around your own learning needs. Never be afraid to ask. They are there to help you!

Why is inhaler technique so important?

There are many different types of inhaler devices on the market as discussed in chapter 5. Everyone's ability to use inhalers is different, therefore your nurse will help you to decide which inhaler is more appropriate for your needs. It is so important that your inhaler suits you. If you find it difficult to use and therefore are not using it as required, this will compromise your condition, leading to poorly controlled asthma.

The NHS is continually reviewing the cost of all medications including asthma inhalers, therefore they try to push the cheaper inhalers. This is fine, if you can use the device, but if you can't, then a more suitable and sometimes costly inhaler device is more appropriate. The most expensive device is the one that is not used because you cannot use it properly.

Checking that your inhaler is not empty is very important. Many of the inhalers have a dose counter and this tells you when you need to order another prescription. Unfortunately, some of the metered dose aerosol inhalers do not have a dose counter. Even when the drug is long gone, the gas remains so it can feel like you are getting your medication as the treatment fires and tastes the same for a long while after the drug is gone.

How to tell if your inhaler is empty:

- Take the canister out of the inhaler device holder.

- Put the canister into a deep bowl of cold water or a pint glass of cold water.

- If the canister is floating and flat, you only have gas in your inhaler and it is empty.

- If it floats but dips at one end, you have some drug remaining but it is almost empty, therefore you need to order another prescription.

- If the canister sinks to the bottom, it is full of drug.

Afterwards, to dry the canister, wipe dry and leave it to air, away from any heat source. When you are satisfied that it is fully dry, push it back into place in the plastic holder. Fire a dose and now it is ready to use.

What is influenza?

Influenza or flu is a viral infection affecting your airways. It is highly infectious and has an incubation period of one to three days. It is transmitted from one person to the other by what is termed 'droplet infection', meaning that through coughing and sneezing, tiny particles from the respiratory tract of one person can be spread to healthy individuals and inhaled, transmitting the disease.

If you have flu, you can expect to experience:

- Fever and chills.

- Headache and general aches and pains.

- Extreme fatigue or tiredness.

- Dry cough, sore throat, stuffed-up nose.

It is an unpleasant illness, similar to the common cold but in terms of flu, you are generally unwell for much longer, often seven days or longer.

Severe flu can be complicated by meningitis or encephalitis. Flu is more serious for newborn babies, the elderly and those who have long-term conditions such as asthma, diabetes, heart disease, kidney disease and multiple sclerosis.

The flu season is traditionally around December till February, although this can vary. For this reason, the flu clinics that are set up to immunise those at risk are set up in early October.

Flu is more serious for newborn babies, the elderly and those who have long-term conditions such as asthma, diabetes, heart disease, kidney disease and multiple sclerosis.

Why is immunisation against influenza and pneumonia so important?

There is strong evidence to suggest that influenza impacts on the health of asthmatics, and a substantial proportion of adults and children are hospitalised each year due to the effects of flu on asthma. In one- to three-year-olds, not only does influenza cause worsening asthma, but it has been implicated in being the causative factor for hospitalisation due to pneumonia, heart failure and other heart problems. This shows that unfortunately, influenza can have a serious effect on asthma and an increased risk of death as a direct complication of the disease.

Immunisation against flu

Immunisation against flu in the UK for high-risk groups has been recommended since the late 1960s. Pregnant women have more recently been included as one of the at risk groups. The protection that immunisation offers, lasts for about one year but can be less in the elderly.

The World Health Organisation (WHO) looks at which strains of influenza are circulating globally. They then advise the drug companies who manufacture the vaccines. The aim is to offer protection against the top three strains of influenza that are predicted to affect the northern hemisphere. The manufacturing of the vaccines is on a tight schedule due to the short time available once WHO have collaborated with the vaccine manufacturers. For this reason, manufacturers may not be able to respond to unexpectedly high demands on stocks at short notice. The flu clinics are organised months in advance of the flu season, where the orders are taken during the summer. During an unexpected pandemic, supplies are used quickly and replacement can be difficult, as we have seen more recently with the swine flu pandemic.

As the strains are evolving and changing all the time, the vaccines are different each winter. The swine flu vaccine became available in 2009, and the uptake for this important vaccine has been excellent. Due to this, the pandemic spread of H1N1 was controlled quickly. For the first time, in October 2010, the swine flu vaccine was added to the normal seasonal flu vaccine and the campaign was very effective in keeping the disease at bay.

What many people do not realise is that any of the flu vaccines take between 10 and 14 days before they offer protection against the more common flu viruses. If someone who has had the vaccine becomes infected with the flu virus before this protection (seroconversion) occurs, then they may still get flu, as they did not have enough time to become immune.

Considering this, the flu clinics are organised to run from the beginning of October, long before the flu season is expected to begin. If you go for your flu vaccine early, then you should get maximum protection. As asthmatics are deemed to be at risk, they are entitled to the flu vaccine each winter. For children who are under the age of 13 and who are having the vaccine for the first time, they need to have the jab repeated four to six weeks later. This is because their immune systems are immature and they need two vaccines to offer maximum protection. After the first year, the child will only need to have one flu vaccine each winter.

For children who are under the age of 13 and who are having the vaccine for the first time, they need to have the jab repeated four to six weeks later.

The side effects with the flu vaccine are minimal. Normally, you may have a sore upper arm for a couple of days and you may experience some swelling or redness. Also, you can sometimes develop a mild fever and paracetamol will quickly reduce any fever. These side effects only appear for a couple of days, if at all.

Very rarely, someone may experience an allergic reaction to the vaccine. Those known to have an egg allergy should inform the nurse or doctor of this before they administer the vaccine. Also, if you have a fever at the time of vaccination, you will not be able to have the jab and will need to make an alternative appointment when your symptoms have subsided.

Pneumococcal vaccine

Pneumococcal disease is caused by the bacterium named streptococcus pneumoniae or pneumococcus. Again, it is transmitted through droplet infection or direct contact with respiratory secretions during coughing or sneezing. The incubation period is one to three days, and the bacterium may spread into the sinuses (sinusitis) or middle ear (middle ear infection) or lungs (pneumonia) or the brain (meningitis).

Pneumonia particularly affects the very young and the elderly, those who have no spleen and those who have a poor immune system.

The pneumococcal vaccine was introduced in 1992 and was offered to those people deemed at risk. Currently, the pneumococcal vaccine is offered as a one-off vaccine. However, those who are at increased risk, such as those with no spleen or those who are immunosupressed, they are advised to have a booster after ten years.

There are two types of pneumococcal vaccine:

- Pneumococcal polysaccharide vaccine – protects against 23 types and accounts for 96% of cases. Most people take three weeks to achieve immunity following the vaccine. Children under the age of two do not achieve a good response to this vaccine.

- Pneumococcal conjugate vaccine – protects against 13 types. This vaccine offers more effective immunity for the under twos and is offered routinely within the child immunisation programme from the age of two months.

The pneumonia vaccine is very safe and effective and the side effects are similar to the influenza vaccine. The pneumonia vaccine is often offered during the seasonal flu clinics, although it is given throughout the year to those at risk and during routine childhood immunisation.

Summing Up

- Your GP and asthma nurse work together in caring for you and your long-term condition.

- Your asthma reviews are very important. Here you will gain the knowledge, confidence and skills to manage your condition effectively.

- Your nurse will help you to identify your own personal asthma triggers and discuss ways that you may be able to avoid these.

- Always take your inhalers and peak flow meter along to your appointment. Your nurse will then be able to check your technique.

- Self-management planning in the form of a written personal action plan is the key to successfully controlling asthma.

- Immunisation against influenza and pneumonia are very effective in reducing asthma exacerbations in susceptible people. Ask your practice nurse for details.

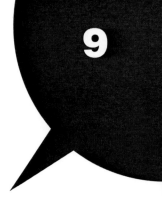

9

Keeping Well

Stepping up and stepping down treatment – what does it mean?

Like many asthmatics, you may have episodes where your asthma is more poorly controlled. However, there can be long periods of time between symptoms, so much so that it can appear that you have 'grown out' of your asthma.

Regular review of patients as treatment is stepped down is important. When deciding which drug to step down first and at what rate, the severity of asthma, the side effects of the treatment, time on current dose, the beneficial effect achieved, and the patient's preference should all be taken into account.

For this reason, you would never be left on a treatment long-term without the offer of regular reviews. If your asthma becomes dormant, meaning that you feel there are no symptoms and do not need to use any inhalers, then your nurse will consider stepping down your treatment to the lowest dose of steroid possible to keep you well controlled. This reduction should be done slowly, for example every three months, decreasing by 25-50% each time. You may be able to come off your steroid inhaler completely.

The BTS/SIGN Guidelines for asthma advises that nurses use a step-wise approach to treating your condition (see Appendix A). These steps are:

Step one

At this step, your asthma is mild and intermittent. You will use your reliever inhaler as often as your require, for example, if you experience shortness of breath, coughing or wheezing or reduced ability to exercise due to these symptoms. You will use your usual reliever as often as is required to relieve these symptoms. If you need to use it more than three or four times per week or at night then you need to move to step two. This is because there will be more inflammation within the airways. The reliever inhaler only relaxes the smooth muscle fibres of the airways and doesn't relieve the inflammation.

Step two

At this step, you will need to add in a regular treatment of inhaled corticosteroid to help relieve the inflammation within the airways. Remember that the preventer inhaler will take a while to become effective, often 10-14 days and in some cases, longer still. When the preventer becomes effective, you will notice that you need to use your reliever less and less. Once your preventer becomes fully active, you should not need to use your reliever very often. If you still need to use your reliever more than three to four times per week, or are still waking sometimes at night, or still have exercise-induced symptoms, then you will probably need to go to step three.

Step three

Here, you may be offered a combination inhaler instead of your preventer. The combination inhaler will have a long-term bronchodilator (lasting 12 hours at a time) and a low dose corticosteroid combined. It will be taken in the morning and at night and should begin to be effective much quicker than a corticosteroid alone. Often, your symptoms can improve within a couple of days. You will still use your reliever when you have your usual asthma symptoms, but you should notice very quickly that your asthma becomes well controlled, allowing you to exercise freely and offering a good night's sleep.

Step four

For those of you who are on maximum combination therapy and still have breakthrough symptoms, you may be offered an anti-leukotriene. This treatment is in addition to your normal treatment and is in the form of a tablet taken at night. This reduces inflammation in a different way to corticosteroids. Some asthmatics may also need to have a tablet called theophylline but this is used rarely now and would be initiated by the doctor normally.

Step five

At this point, you are classed as having severe asthma symptoms which will require, along with your inhalers, a once daily oral steroid tablet at the lowest possible dose to achieve control.

For those asthmatics who are difficult to control and who need regularly to be treated at step four to five, they may be sent to their local chest clinic for continuing assessment and review.

While your treatment is being adjusted, you will be monitored regularly. Once you become well controlled, it is advisable to continue on that step of treatment for at least three months before you start to reduce your therapy. Always listen to the advice of your doctor or nurse.

It is a good idea to write any questions down that you may want to ask your doctor or nurse, so that you don't forget.

It is a good idea to write any questions down that you may want to ask your doctor or nurse, so that you don't forget. Always take your inhalers and any asthma diaries with you to your appointment.

Always take your inhalers and any asthma diaries with you to your appointment.

How will I know that my asthma is poorly controlled?

Remember (as explained in chapter 7) the signs that show that your asthma is less well controlled are:

- Waking at night with shortness of breath, wheezing or coughing and needing to use your reliever inhaler.

- Needing to use more reliever treatment, or the treatment doesn't seem to work for as long as usual.

- Waking up earlier than usual due to asthma symptoms.

- A fall in your peak flow readings or maybe a wide difference between your peak flow readings on waking, compared to those in the evening.

- Unusual breathlessness when exerting yourself or when exercising.

- Reduced ability to perform your usual activities due to asthma symptoms.

These signs are showing that you need to see your doctor or nurse to have your treatment reviewed. You may need some other therapy to gain quick and effective control of your symptoms. Make your appointment to see your doctor or nurse now.

If, as shown in chapter 7, you have the following symptoms:

- Too breathless to talk.

- Your peak flow reading is 50% or less of your usual readings.

- Your reliever inhaler is not working.

You need to re-visit chapter 7, where page 68 will remind you what to do.

If you feel your asthma is poorly controlled but not at danger point, then you need to book an urgent appointment with your doctor or nurse. Always stress to the reception staff that your asthma is out of control and that you need an urgent appointment. If you do not tell them it is out of control, they may not offer you an appointment for a few days, which could mean that your asthma becomes very much worse.

What is airway remodelling?

As previously mentioned, asthma is an inflammatory condition of the airways. Alterations of the structure to the tissues within the airways, known as 'remodelling' can occur as a response to chronic inflammation of the airways. This shows in the form of muscle wall thickening through muscle swelling, (in fatal asthma there can be a 50-300% increase) increased mucus secretion, myofibroblast hyperplasia, and abnormalities to the normal blood supply of the lungs.

In normal health, we know that our lung function declines with age over time. Unfortunately, asthmatics can experience a more accelerated rate of lung function deterioration. Also, remodelling can permanently alter the normal tissue function, leading to irreversible damage and a more rapidly declining lung function.

In fatal asthma, the airways have been found to have increased smooth muscle fibres, leading to increased swelling, and complete obstruction of the airways due to viscous or sticky mucus plugs.

For this reason, it is so important that you make the most of the help that is offered to you and that you try and gain the best control of your symptoms. We know that asthma is termed a 'variable' disease, meaning that you can have episodes of normal lung function. But we also know that if you have poorly controlled asthma, then this can cause life-long damage due to the persistent inflammation and swelling of the airways. In the worst case scenario, it can cause death.

Using a peak flow meter

As mentioned in chapter 5, peak flow meters are portable hand-held devices which we use to measure how much you can blow out of your lungs in one, quick, fast blow. The ability to blow out depends on how symptomatic you are at that present time. If your asthma is not troublesome, your peak flow will be at its best, but if you are troubled by your symptoms the result can vary considerably.

A peak flow meter is available in two ranges, one for small children and one for older children, teenagers and adults. There are several differing designs on the market currently. Your nurse or doctor can help you decide which one better suits your needs.

If you regularly need to change your inhaler therapy, then a peak flow meter can be of real benefit.

Remember, that a wide variation between your morning and evening peak flow can show that your asthma is out of control. Book an appointment with your asthma nurse.

If you take your peak flow readings and your asthma diary with you to your appointment, the nurse will be able to help you to develop an asthma action plan to suit your personal needs.

Travel – thinking ahead

Excitement of a holiday and a new environment may trigger your asthma symptoms.

Even though you may feel well and have not been troubled by your asthma for a while, if you are going away on holiday or abroad, you will need to be prepared. Out of your normal environment, your triggers may change and you may become unstable while away.

Remember, that a wide variation between your morning and evening peak flow can show that your asthma is out of control.

- Ensure you have plenty of supplies of your usual inhaled medication.

- If you have had severe symptoms in the past, check with your nurse if you need a short course of rescue therapy – oral prednisolone – to take with you just in case of an emergency.

- Carry your reliever inhaler in your hand luggage.

- Remember, if you are holidaying in the UK, you can be seen as a temporary resident at any surgery. Contact NHS Direct who will be able to give you details of your local doctor's surgery while you are away.

- If pets or cigarette smoke are one of your triggers, request a room that has not been used for smokers or pets.

- Ensure your travel insurance company knows you have asthma.

- Check and see if you need a letter from your doctor that states you are fit to travel.

- Travel insurance for asthmatics can be found by accessing Asthma UK (see help list). There is no age limit and Asthma UK will receive a donation per policy sold.

What is the role of rescue therapy?

Remember that if you have ever had a severe asthma exacerbation, your doctor or nurse may have given you a prescription for a spare course of steroid tablets, to be taken in the event that your asthma becomes very severe. Generally, if your peak flow readings are 50% or lower of your usual best, and your normal reliever medication seems not to be effective, it is time to use your rescue therapy. Take it as soon as you are worried but remember to book an appointment with a doctor or nurse as soon as you can, preferably on the same day. Remember, even if your symptoms improve over the course of the day, you could get a much worse episode during the night.

Lifestyle advice

If your peak flow readings are 50% or lower of your usual best, and your normal reliever medication seems not to be effective, it is time to use your rescue therapy.

The British Guideline on the Management of Asthma indicates that studies show that if you gain weight which increases your body mass index, then this can have an effect of worsening your asthma symptoms. This highlights the point of aiming for a body mass index of between 20 and 25. Your nurse can help you with dietary advice.

Remember, as detailed in chapter 6, that tobacco smoke is an irritant which inflames and irritates the airways and can contribute to worsening your symptoms. Also, mothers who smoke during pregnancy can increase the risk of their babies developing asthma symptoms. Any exposure to cigarette smoke can affect your quality of life, your lung function and your more frequent need for oral steroid rescue therapy. Again, your nurse will have the skills to help you to reduce or stop smoking altogether. Alternatively, you could access any of the help resources as listed in the help list at the back of this book.

Exercise is important to us all but in terms of asthma, especially if you have needed to rely on short courses of oral steroids, then exercise will help reduce your risk of developing osteoporosis in later life. This can be a consequence of frequent or prolonged oral steroids.

Allergen avoidance

Being able to identify your own personal triggers is very useful. You may not be able to avoid them completely but trigger reduction can help. For example, if you know that grass pollen affects you, then you could avoid cutting the grass, whilst keeping the windows shut. Also, knowing that your triggers are seasonal can alert you to stepping up your treatment in advance which will reduce your risk of unwanted symptoms.

Ensure that your home is well ventilated and clear of moulds and spores. It is amazing how a little mould in your bathroom can affect your asthma. Also, bought compost can contain moulds. The best time to garden is in the morning on a fine sunny day. By evening, as the temperature drops, so does the pollen, so avoid evening gardening. Close all windows prior to and during thunderstorms for allergen avoidance.

Remember that hay fever and rhinitis can co-exist with asthma. You can control your hay fever symptoms by going along to your local pharmacy where they can offer you a selection of therapies including antihistamines, nasal steroids and eye drops.

Pre-Payment Certificates

At times, asthma treatments can be very costly and this can have an implication on your symptoms if you cannot afford your treatment. If you pay for four or more prescriptions every three months, a Pre-Payment Certificate may save you a lot of money.

You can access one of these by:

- Phoning 0845 850 0030.
- Using the NHS's online application form.
- Asking at your local pharmacy.
- Asking for details at your GPs surgery.

Staying away from home overnight

If you or your child sleeps elsewhere at night, for example at their grandparents' home, or maybe your child is co-parented, it is very important that other carers are up to date with their asthma skills and knowledge. It is important that parents and grandparents are fully informed as to what to do during an attack and how the specific treatments work. Your nurse would be more than happy for these carers to attend at your child's asthma review.

If your child is symptomatic when they are due to sleep elsewhere, it is probably best that this is avoided, especially if it is at a friend's house. At best it would be unfair to your child and to the other family. At worst, your child will be at risk if his/her symptoms worsen. Remember that symptoms generally worsen during the middle of the night.

If your child regularly has sleepovers with other members of the family, ask your nurse for more inhalers so that they can be left behind.

Summing Up

- Your doctor or nurse will treat your asthma using a step-wise approach to therapy and will wish to review you regularly.

- Remember to book an appointment with your nurse as soon as you notice your symptoms are bothering you more than three times a week or if you are waking due to your asthma.

- Due to chronic inflammation as a result of poor control, the structures in your airways can re-model, resulting in irreversible damage to your airways.

- A peak flow meter is a useful device which helps you to monitor your symptom control effectively.

- When travelling or sleeping away from home, make sure you have enough of your medications. A new environment can trigger your symptoms.

- A healthy lifestyle which includes plenty of exercise, optimal weight control and not being exposed to cigarette smoke can help control your asthma.

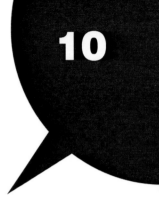

10

Additional Information

Can complementary therapies help?

There is some evidence to suggest that complementary therapies can have a beneficial effect on asthma. These include herbal remedies, aromatherapy, homeopathy, reflexology, acupuncture and acupressure.

- The Buteyko breathing control technique claims to have a positive effect on asthma. It is a system of breathing exercises, and behavioural changes which are said to balance the oxygen and carbon dioxide levels in exhaled air. Buteyko technique is claimed to help people adapt to their asthma symptoms. Currently, there is no research to back this claim up.

- Yoga uses a variety of postures and breathing techniques to improve fitness and to help with relaxation. Studies have shown that a form of yoga called pranayama exercises has been found to be beneficial by reducing the number of exacerbations and increasing tolerance to triggers.

- Hypnotherapy involves techniques to create a state of decreased general awareness which allows someone to concentrate wholly on one particular thing or idea. However, not everyone is susceptible to hypnosis.

- Acupuncture involves the insertion of fine sterile needles at specific sites of the body which are claimed to balance the body's natural energy meridians, offering short-term benefits to asthmatics. It is said that it is of more use to those with allergic asthma rather that exercise-induced asthma.

- Homeopathy involves preparing medicines which include traces of the substance to which a person is allergic to, for example pollens or dust mites. Homeopathic immunotherapy has been shown through research to help with asthma and rhinitis symptoms.

- Herbal remedies are one of the oldest known form of medicines in the modern world. However, there is little evidence to show that it is beneficial. In fact the herbal remedy named St. John's wort has been found to reduce the effect of the medication theophylline, which is sometimes used from step three of the Asthma Guidelines upwards. Royal jelly and propolis (bee glue) have been found to have very serious side effects in asthmatics, resulting in severe allergic reactions, including death.

There is some evidence to suggest that complementary therapies can have a beneficial effect on asthma.

For more information on complementary therapies and what they entail, take a look at *Complementary Therapies – The Essential Guide* (Need2Know).

'The main complementary therapies that can help your asthma are, aromatherapy, herbal medicine, naturopathy, homeopathy, osteopathy, chiropractic, reflexology, Rolfing, Alexander Technique, acupuncture and breath control techniques.'

Dr Sarah Brewer – Natural Health Guru – *Overcoming Asthma – the complete complementary health program*. (2009)

Can a nutritional approach help to control my asthma?

There is strong evidence to suggest that some foods can have either a positive or negative effect on asthma.

To improve your symptoms, evidence suggests that you should increase:

- Omega 3s found in oily fish such as herring, mackerel, tuna, salmon and sardines. Eat more nuts, and take Omega 3 supplements.

- Fruit and vegetables, especially dark green vegetables.

To improve your symptoms, evidence suggests that you should reduce or stop:

- Omega 6, which is important for hormonal control, it needs to be used sparingly so reduce vegetable oils.

- Meat, which contain proteins known to cause allergies. Meat-eaters tend to produce more leukotrienes which have an inflammatory effect on the airways. It would be better to eat meat only three times per week.

- Salt intake. This can encourage fluid retention which has been found to increase congestion in the lung tissue causing constriction.

- Any foods that you believe may impact on your asthma. This could include milk, eggs, peanuts, citrus fruits, food additives and wheat.

- Margarine.

- Fast food and processed food, including pastries, biscuits and cakes.

What are salicylates and how can they affect my asthma?

Acetylsalicylic acid, more commonly known as aspirin, has been used for years to treat pain and fever. It has been suggested that many asthmatics have their symptoms triggered by aspirin or foodstuffs containing salicylates, especially those aged between 20-40.

Acetylsalicylic acid, more commonly known as aspirin, has been used for years to treat pain and fever. It has been suggested that many asthmatics have their symptoms triggered by aspirin or foodstuffs containing salicylates, especially those aged between 20-40. These triggers can sometimes cause a severe attack. If you are aware that you are allergic to salicylates, you need to avoid all food and medicines containing salicylate. Salicylate allergy can also cause allergic rhinitis, nasal polyps and allergic sinusitis, and can contribute to a loss of smell.

This also means that you should avoid non-steroidal, anti-inflammatory drugs such as ibuprofen, naproxen, diclofenac and meloxicam, as they can trigger an attack in those who are aspirin-sensitive.

Salicylate-laden foods include:

- Asparagus, aubergine, avocado, broccoli, cucumber, Granny Smith apples, grapefruit, peach, potatoes, squash, spinach watercress.

- Herbs and spices such as aniseed, cayenne, cinnamon, celery seed, cumin, cloves, curry powder, dill, ginger, liquorice, mace, marjoram, mint, mustard seed, oregano, pepper, sage, tarragon, thyme, turmeric, basil, tea leaves, white pepper, chicory.

- Currants, dates, prunes, raisins, raspberries, apricots, oranges, pineapple, almonds, cantaloupe melon, cranberries, grapes, green peppers and olives, courgettes, peanuts, radishes, strawberries.

- Other flavourings such as stock cubes, Worcestershire sauce, yeast extracts, vanilla essence.

- Drinks, including wine, champagne, coffee, tea.

Salicylate-free foods include:

- Bamboo shoots, bean sprouts, beetroot, celery, green cabbage, split peas, bananas, black eye beans, chickpeas, lima beans, mung beans, soy beans, split peas, poppy seeds, gin, vodka and whisky, camomile tea, malt vinegar.

What about tartrazine?

Tartrazine is an artificial yellow food colouring which is produced synthetically. Since the 1970s, it has been required that tartrazine levels are identified through food labelling. Some toiletries and cosmetics also contain tartrazine.

Tartrazine-containing foods have been shown to trigger asthma symptoms. If you have too much tartrazine, it causes a release of histamine from mast cells in your airways.

Foods containing tartrazine include biscuits, cereals, cakes, cake mixes, crisps, crackers, chocolates, fizzy drinks, mixer drinks, cordials and fruit cocktails, some food sauces, mustards, processed meats and fish, smoked cod and haddock, vitamin and mineral supplements, processed cheeses, custards and custard powders and ready-made desserts.

For many reasons, it is a good idea to get into the habit of checking all food labels before purchase and to try and enjoy home cooking.

What is the 'Smart System'?

AstraZenica has recently launched the 'Smart System' which is a newer approach to asthma management. Although not mentioned in the current BTS/SIGN Guidelines, their drug therapy, Symbicort, can be used for daily maintenance therapy and also used in addition when relief of symptoms is required. Symbicort is a combination inhaler therapy which contains the inhaled corticosteroid budesonide combined with a long-acting bronchodilator, formoterol. It is normally used at step three of the BTS/SIGN Guidelines. It is considered for use for those who are inadequately controlled and frequently require their reliever inhaler.

This method of therapy requires frequent, close monitoring with either an asthma nurse or a GP. Anyone on the 'Smart System' can get dose-related side effects, particularly if whilst on this system, they still require frequent relieving doses.

The Smart System is not licensed for those under the age of 18. Currently, there is no adequate data regarding use in pregnancy or lactation. A risk/benefit analysis would have to be made in these circumstances.

What are Xolair injections?

Xolair is a new add-on therapy for those asthmatics who, despite regular maintenance therapy, suffer severe day and night symptoms with frequent exacerbations. Xolair is given in injection form, 1-4 injections, given either at two or four weekly intervals.

Xolair is a man-made protein which works by blocking immunoglobulin E (IgE), a substance produced by our bodies that causes the allergic reaction. It can take between 12 and 16 weeks to become effective.

This treatment should not be used in those under the age of six, or pregnant ladies or those who are breastfeeding. This therapy requires special monitoring and is not usually started by your GP. Most asthmatics on this therapy would be monitored at a special chest clinic.

Xolair is a new add-on therapy for those asthmatics who despite regular maintenance therapy, suffer severe day and night symptoms with frequent exacerbations.

What is Bronchial thermoplasty?

This is a very new and exciting therapy currently undergoing tests. It provides relief for those with mild to moderate asthma, who do not respond to conventional asthma therapy, offering more symptom-free days and better control of triggers.

Performed on an outpatient basis, this treatment involves a light anaesthesia. A flexible tube called a bronchoscope is passed through the nose or mouth, into the airways and a catheter is passed through, which sends radio frequency energy to the side of the airway wall. This heats the smooth muscle wall to 149°F, with the effect of thinning and weakening the muscle, without causing damage or scarring. The result is that the muscle wall cannot then contract fully when a further attack occurs. Currently, five pilot sites are using this technique.

Summing Up

- Complementary therapies such as acupuncture, aromatherapy, reflexology, homeopathy, yoga, and Buteyko breathing exercises claim to have a beneficial effect on asthma.

- Interestingly, many foods can have either a positive or negative effect on your asthma symptoms.

- Salicylate (aspirin) which is naturally occurring in foods, as well as found in some medicines, can trigger asthma in those who are susceptible.

- Tartrazine, a yellow food colouring can also trigger symptoms.

- Newer strategies at controlling asthma involve the 'Smart System' – using a combination inhaler both for regular maintenance therapy as well as reliever therapy.

- Xolair is an injection sometimes used for those with severe allergic asthma, but it is given usually under strict control and is not a common therapy for asthma.

- Bronchial thermoplasty is a new therapy currently undergoing tests. It is performed as a day case under a light anaesthetic.

Glossary

Airway remodelling
This is where the tissue structures of the airways are altered. This can occur due to chronic inflammation. During this process, the smooth muscle thickens and swells. There is increased mucus production and there are changes to the normal blood supply to the tissues. This change can become permanent.

Allergens
Any substance that can cause an allergic reaction. This could be house dust mite, cigarette smoke, moulds, perfumes, pollens, animal dander, food additives. The list is endless.

Allergy testing
This is used to identify allergies and takes the form of a detailed history, combined with skin prick testing and blood testing.

Atopy
A condition which triggers an allergic reaction when there is exposure to an allergen.

Combination therapy
Combination inhalers which contain both preventers and protectors. Research shows that given in combination offers a better therapeutic effect.

Compliance
Refers to the ability or willingness of someone in taking prescribed medication or following a treatment plan.

Exacerbation
Describes a sudden asthma attack or steadily worsening symptoms.

Inspiratory flow rate
This refers to the speed at which someone can breathe in their drug therapy using an inhaler.

Leukotriene receptor antagonist
Tablets taken at night to help reduce inflammation, often triggered by allergens and exercise.

Neurological changes
Term that describes alteration in normal brain function.

Occupational asthma
This describes symptoms that are triggered by exposure in the workplace.

Passive smoking
Refers to when we inhale second-hand smoke from other people's cigarettes.

Peak expiratory flow rate
This is measured using a peak flow meter which identifies the severity of obstruction within the airways.

Preventers (corticosteroids)

Very low dose inhaled drug therapy which reduce inflammation within the tissues of the lungs, thereby controlling asthma symptoms. There is a slow onset of action when using these inhaled drugs.

Protectors (long-acting bronchodilators)

Inhaled drug therapy which works by relaxing the bronchial smooth muscle. This relieves spasm but it takes a while for the effect to begin. These drugs work for 12 hours at a time.

Relievers (bronchodilators)

Inhaled drug therapy which relaxes the smooth muscle fibres of the airways. This effect is immediate.

Rescue therapy

This takes the form of a short course of steroid tablets, to be taken if your asthma suddenly becomes worse, particularly if your peak flow is 50% or less than your normal reading.

Reversibility testing

A diagnostic procedure using lung function equipment to identify variations in airflow obstruction; the results of which can be used to form a diagnosis of asthma.

Self-management plan

Through education and support from your nurse or doctor, you can develop a personal action plan which will help you to manage your condition more effectively.

Spirometry

Lung function testing equipment often used at your GPs surgery. It can be used to perform reversibility testing.

Trigger

Any substance which causes the symptoms of asthma.

Variability

This is found during lung function testing and describes the wide variations of obstruction between your good and bad days. The wider the variability, the more poorly controlled the asthma.

Appendix A

Summary of stepwise management in adults
Image courtesy the British Theracic Society

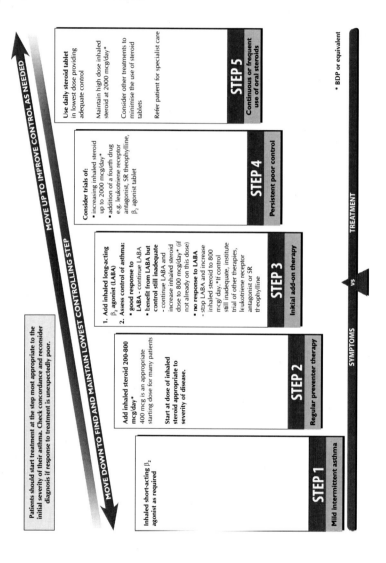

MOVE UP TO IMPROVE CONTROL AS NEEDED

MOVE DOWN TO FIND AND MAINTAIN LOWEST CONTROLLING STEP

Patients should start treatment at the step most appropriate to the initial severity of their asthma. Check concordance and reconsider diagnosis if response to treatment is unexpectedly poor.

STEP 1
Mild intermittent asthma

Inhaled short-acting β_2 agonist as required

STEP 2
Regular preventer therapy

Add inhaled steroid 200-800 mcg/day*

400 mcg is an appropriate starting dose for many patients

Start at dose of inhaled steroid appropriate to severity of disease.

STEP 3
Initial add-on therapy

1. Add inhaled long-acting β_2 agonist (LABA)
2. Assess control of asthma:
   - **good response to LABA** - continue LABA
   - **benefit from LABA but control still inadequate** - continue LABA and increase inhaled steroid dose to 800 mcg/day* (if not already on this dose)
   - **no response to LABA** - stop LABA and increase inhaled steroid to 800 mcg/day. *If control still inadequate, institute trial of other therapies, leukotriene receptor antagonist or SR theophylline

STEP 4
Persistent poor control

Consider trials of:
- increasing inhaled steroid up to 2000 mcg/day*
- addition of a fourth drug e.g. leukotriene receptor antagonist, SR theophylline, β_2 agonist tablet

STEP 5
Continuous or frequent use of oral steroids

Use daily steroid tablet in lowest dose providing adequate control

Maintain high dose inhaled steroid at 2000 mcg/day*

Consider other treatments to minimise the use of steroid tablets

Refer patient for specialist care

SYMPTOMS vs TREATMENT

* BDP or equivalent

Summary of stepwise management in children aged 5-12 years

Image courtesy the British Theracic Society

Patients should start treatment at the step most appropriate to the initial severity of their asthma. Check concordance and reconsider diagnosis if response to treatment is unexpectedly poor.

MOVE UP TO IMPROVE CONTROL AS NEEDED

MOVE DOWN TO FIND AND MAINTAIN LOWEST CONTROLLING STEP

STEP 1
Mild intermittent asthma

Inhaled short-acting β_2 agonist as required

STEP 2
Regular preventer therapy

Add inhaled steroid 200-400 mcg/day* (other preventer drug if inhaled steroid cannot be used) 200 mcg is an appropriate starting dose for many patients

Start at dose of inhaled steroid appropriate to severity of disease.

STEP 3
Initial add-on therapy

1. Add inhaled long-acting β_2 agonist (LABA)
2. Assess control of asthma:
   - **good response to LABA**
     - continue LABA
   - **benefit from LABA but control still inadequate**
     - continue LABA and increase inhaled steroid dose to 400 mcg/day* (if not already on this dose)
   - **no response to LABA**
     - stop LABA and increase inhaled steroid to 400 mcg/ day. *If control still inadequate, institute trial of other therapies, leukotriene receptor antagonist or SR theophylline

STEP 4
Persistent poor control

Increase inhaled steroid up to 800 mcg/day*

STEP 5
Continuous or frequent use of oral steroids

Use daily steroid tablet in lowest dose providing adequate control

Maintain high dose inhaled steroid at 800 mcg/day*

Refer to respiratory paediatrician

SYMPTOMS vs TREATMENT

* BDP or equivalent

Summary of stepwise management in children less than 5 years
Image courtesy the British Theracic Society

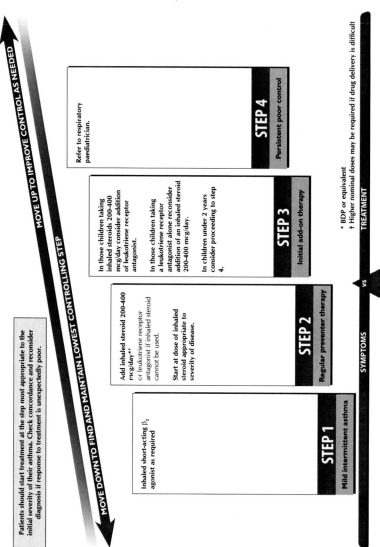

MOVE UP TO IMPROVE CONTROL AS NEEDED

MOVE DOWN TO FIND AND MAINTAIN LOWEST CONTROLLING STEP

Patients should start treatment at the step most appropriate to the initial severity of their asthma. Check concordance and reconsider diagnosis if response to treatment is unexpectedly poor.

STEP 1
Mild intermittent asthma

Inhaled short-acting β₂ agonist as required

STEP 2
Regular preventer therapy

Add inhaled steroid 200-400 mcg/day**†**
or leukotriene receptor antagonist if inhaled steroid cannot be used.

Start at dose of inhaled steroid appropriate to severity of disease.

STEP 3
Initial add-on therapy

In those children taking inhaled steroids 200-400 mcg/day consider addition of leukotriene receptor antagonist.

In those children taking a leukotriene receptor antagonist alone reconsider addition of an inhaled steroid 200-400 mcg/day.

In children under 2 years consider proceeding to step 4.

STEP 4
Persistent poor control

Refer to respiratory paediatrician.

SYMPTOMS — vs — TREATMENT

* BDP or equivalent
† Higher nominal doses may be required if drug delivery is difficult

Appendix B

asthma action plan

name

name of doctor/nurse

contact number for surgery

Image courtesy Chiesi Ltd

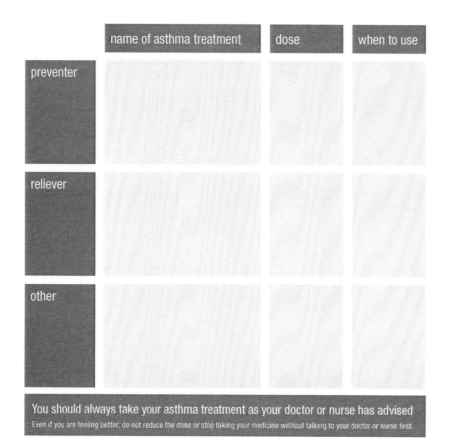

	name of asthma treatment	dose	when to use
preventer			
reliever			
other			

You should always take your asthma treatment as your doctor or nurse has advised
Even if you are feeling better, do not reduce the dose or stop taking your medicine without talking to your doctor or nurse first.

Image courtesy Chiesi Ltd

need2know

review these questions regularly

This will help you to recognise if your asthma symptoms are getting worse.[1]

Have you had difficulty sleeping because of your asthma symptoms (including coughing)?

Have you had your usual asthma symptoms during the day (wheezing, coughing, shortness of breath, tightness in the chest)?

Has your asthma interfered with your usual activities (e.g. housework, work or school)?

If you answer yes to one or more of these questions, or if you haven't had your asthma reviewed for twelve months or more, arrange to see your doctor or nurse.

If your asthma gets worse:
If your symptoms do not improve after ___ days, contact your doctor or nurse.

what to do if you have an asthma attack:

If you have an asthma attack, you should call a doctor, 999, or go to hospital immediately.

Reference: 1. Asthma UK. Controlling your asthma. Available at: www.asthma.org.uk/all_about_asthma/controlling_your_asthma/index. html. Date accessed April 2010.

Date of preparation: APRIL 2010 I Job code: WEL20100001

Image courtesy Chiesi Ltd

Appendix C

How to record your peak flow in your diary

You should record your peak flow twice a day – once in the morning and once in the evening. See the last page of your diary for instructions on how to use your peak flow meter.

To record your peak flow, mark an 'X' on the chart for that day under AM or PM, depending on when you are taking your measurement. You might also find it helpful to connect the X's with a line – you will see a line graph emerging that will show you at a glance how your peak flow may be getting better, worse or staying the same over time.

It is also a good idea to keep track of any asthma symptoms you might be experiencing as it is easy to forget these later. You can record this by circling yes or no on each of the three questions every day. There is also a space to record the number of times you use your reliever inhaler every day. Keeping track of your symptoms is also useful for your doctor or asthma nurse so that they can see how well controlled your asthma is on your next visit.

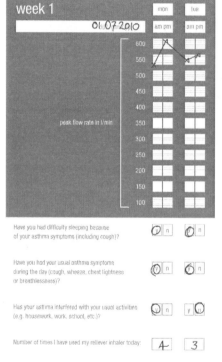

Image courtesy Chiesi Ltd

week 1

dd / mm / yy

	mon	tue	wed	thu	fri	sat	sun
	am pm	am pm	am pm	am pm	am pm	am pm	am pm

peak flow rate in l/min

600
550
500
450
400
350
300
250
200
150
100

Have you had difficulty sleeping because of your asthma symptoms (including cough)?
y n   y n   y n   y n   y n   y n   y n

Have you had your usual asthma symptoms during the day (cough, wheeze, chest tightness or breathlessness)?
y n   y n   y n   y n   y n   y n   y n

Has your asthma interfered with your usual activities (e.g. housework, work, school, etc.)?
y n   y n   y n   y n   y n   y n   y n

Number of times I have used my reliever inhaler today:

Image courtesy Chiesi Ltd

How to use your peak flow meter

The meter has a pointer that slides
up the scale as you blow out. To take a
peak flow reading, follow these instructions:

1. Check that the pointer is at the bottom of the scale

2. Preferably stand or sit in a comfortable, upright position

3. Hold the peak flow meter level (horizontally)
   and keep your fingers away from the pointer

4. Take a deep breath and close your lips firmly
   around the mouthpiece

5. Blow as hard as you can

6. Look at the pointer and make a note of your reading

7. Reset the pointer back to the bottom of the scale

To record your peak flow, take three readings
at each time and write down your highest score.
You should record your best peak flow score twice a day
(morning and night, ideally at the same time each day).

Image courtesy Chiesi Ltd

Help List

Action on Smoking and Heath (ASH)
Address: 6th floor, Suites 59-63, New House, 67-68 Hatton Garden, London, EC1N 8JY
Tel: 0207 404 0242 | Email: enquiries@ash.org.uk
Website: http://ash.org.uk/
Info: ASH is a campaigning public health charity that works to eliminate the harm caused by tobacco.

Allergy UK
Address: Planwell House, LEFA Business Park, Edgington Way, Sidcup, Kent DA14 5BH
Tel: 01322619898 | Email: info@allergyuk.org
Website: http://www.allergyuk.org/
Info: Website gives free advice on allergies and intolerances generally.

Asthma UK
Address: 18 Mansell Street London E1 8AA
Tel: 0300 222 5800 | Email: info@asthma.org.uk
Website: https://www.asthma.org.uk
Info@ Asthma UK are an organisation that seek to alleviate the effects of asthma and ultimately cure asthma. Useful website for finding ways to help, e.g. volunteering or donating.

Asthma UK Centre for Applied Research
Address: Usher Institute, University of Edinburgh, Old Medical School, Teviot Place, Edinburgh, EH8 9AG
Email: aukcar.admin@ed.ac.uk
Website: http://www.aukcar.ac.uk/
Info: An exciting new venture between Asthma UK, leading asthma researchers from universities across the UK, people affected by asthma, NHS partners and other organisations. At the forefront of research into asthma.

British Complementary Medicine Association (BCMA)
Address: PO Box 5122, Bournemouth, BH8 OWG
Tel: 0845 3455 977 | Email: office@bcma.co.uk
Website: http://www.bcma.co.uk/
Info: Provides information on various complementary or/supplementary therapies for asthma, among other things.

British Lung Foundation

Address: 73-75 Goswell Road, London, EC1V 7ER
Tel: 020 7688 5555 | Email: Contact form available at https://www.blf.org.uk/get-in-touch#email
Website: https://www.blf.org.uk
Info: Charity with general interest in lung health, clean air, etc.

British Thoracic Society

Address: The British Thoracic Society, 17 Doughty St, London, WC1N 2PL
Tel: 020 7831 8778 | Email: bts@brit-thoracic.org.uk
Website: https://www.brit-thoracic.org.uk/
Info: The BTS is an organisation of doctors and other professionals with an academic interest in asthma- their website has a Learning Hub with various relevant online courses.

Buteyko Breathing Association

Address: 15 Stanley Place, Chipping Ongar, Essex, CM5 9SU
Email: info@buteykobreathing.org
Website: www.buteykobreathing.org/
Info: Non-profit organisation which provides free information and resources on the Buteyko breathing technique, an alternative physical therapy which some people with asthma find useful.

Education for Health and Respiratory Education UK

Address: The Athenaeum/10 Church St, Warwick, CV34 4AB
Tel: 01926 493313 | Email: info@educationforhealth.org
Website: https://www.educationforhealth.org
Info: Education for Health incorporates Respiratory Education UK, which offers a Masters Programme specifically for those interested in learning more about the respiratory system.

Health and Safety Executive

Address: Phase 1, Ty Glas Road, Llanishen, Cardiff CF14 5SH
Tel: 029 2026 3000 | Email: http://www.hse.gov.uk/contact/contact.htm
Website: http://www.hse.gov.uk/
Info: For those who have asthma symptoms related to their workplace.

The National Institute for Occupational Safety and Health

Address: 1600 Clifton Road Atlanta, GA 30329-4027 USA
Tel: +141-800-232-4636 | Email: general@niosh.com
Website: http://www.cdc.gov/niosh/
Info: Another useful organisation for those interested in how their occupation can trigger and worsen their asthma.

No Smoking Day

Address: 59 Redchurch Street, London, E2 7DJ

Tel: 020 7739 5110 | Email: mail@nosmokingday.org.uk

Website: https://www.nosmokingday.org.uk/

Info: No Smoking Day is an annual health awareness day in the U.K. which is intended to help smokers who want to quit. Get involved through the website.

Primary Care Respiratory Society

Address: PCRS-UK, Unit 2, Warwick House, Kingsbury Road, Curdworth, Warwickshire, B76 9EE

Tel: 01675 477600 | Email: info@pcrs-uk.org

Website: https://www.pcrs-uk.org

Info: A professional society which seeks to influence government policy in the UK.

QUIT

Address: 63 St Mary's Axe, London, EC3A 8AA

Tel: 0800 002 200 ('Quitline') | Email: stopsmoking@quit.org.uk

Website: www.quit.org.uk

Info: Quit is the foremost charity organisation for those who want to quit smoking. Useful resource with hints and tips on quitting, as well as resources for groups one can join.

World Allergy Organisation

Address: WAO Secretariat, 555 East Wells Street, Suite 1100, Milwaukee, W1 53202-3823, USA

Tel: +14142761791 | Email: info@worldallergy.org

Website: http://www.worldallergy.org/

Info: WAO collaborating with member societies to provide direct educational outreach programs, symposia and lectureships to members in nearly 100 countries around the globe. One of the foremost authorities on asthma and other allergies.

Book List

Asthma: The Facts
Arshad, S.H. (Oxford University Press, 2008)

Understanding Asthma
Ayres, J. (Family Doctor Publications Ltd, 2008)

Asthma For Dummies
Berger, W. (For Dummies, 2004)

Overcoming Asthma – the Complete Complementary Health Program
Brewer, S. (Duncan Baird Publishers, 2009)

Asthma Allergies, Children: A Parent's Guide
Ehrlich, P. (Third Avenue Books, 2010)

The Asthma Educator's Handbook
Fanta, C.H., et al. (McGraw-Hill Education, 2007)

Global Initiative for Asthma, 2016 Pocket Guide for Asthma Management and Prevention: For Adults and Children Older than 5 Years
(CreateSpace, 2016)

Asthma: Rapid Reference Series
Levy, M.L., ct al. (Rapid Reference, 2004)

Combat Asthma Through Diet
McConville, B. (Southwater, 2009)

Breathe To Heal: Break Free From Asthma
Yakovleva, S. (Breathing Center, 2016)

References and Bibliography

Allen & Hanbury's *Action Asthma; get going with confidence*. 2005

D.E. Dulek, R.S. Peebles, *Viruses and asthma, Biochim. Biophys*. Acta (2011), doi:10.1016/j. bbagen.2011.01.012

Diagnosing Childhood Asthma in Primary Care, found at www.webmentorlibrary.com on 18.10.10

DOH. (2006) *Immunisation against infectious disease* TSO, Third edition

Elias JA. *Airway Remodeling in Asthma. Unanswered Questions* – Section of Pulmonary and critical Care Medicine, Yale University School of Medicine, New Havel, Connecticut. Vol 161. pp S168-S171, 2000

Management of Adult Asthma, found at www.webmentorlibrary.com accessed on 18.10.10

Management of childhood asthma, Pulse published by MSD.Sept 2008

NICE Chronic Obstructive Pulmonary Disease, Guidelines 12 June 2010

Skold CM. *Remodeling in asthma and COPD – differences and similarities*. Clin Respir J 2010; 4 (Suppl. 1): 20-27

Smith DR A, *Illustrated pocketbook of asthma*. The Parthenon Publishing Group INC.2001

The British Thoracic Society Scottish intercollegiate guidelines network. *British Guideline on the Management of Asthma, Quick reference guide*. May 2008

Thorax – an international journal of respiratory medicine. *British Guideline on the management of asthma*. BMJ 2003